Table of Contents

Sommario

Introduction

Ketogenic Diet

Very few carbohydrates, tons of fats, tons of proteins: these are the essential principles of the ketogenic diet, an eating regimen that has become increasingly popular as a diet to reduce. There are many variants of the keto diet, which is extremely fashionable today, all sharing the common feature of cutting carbohydrates as a "trick" to form the body use fats as fuel rather than them, with the results of losing weight.

Ketogenic diet: what's it?

The ketogenic diet may be a dietary regimen that gives a really low intake of carbohydrates and a high content of protein and, above all, fat.

The drastic reduction of carbohydrates in favor of other nutrients aims to force the body to use fats as a source of energy, to market weight loss. The name "ketogenic" derives from the very fact that this diet, by drastically reducing the intake of carbohydrates, results in the formation of the so-called ketone bodies.

History

The ketogenic diet began as a low-carbohydrate eating plan aimed toward reducing seizures in patients who didn't answer medication, especially in children. Very low carbohydrate diets are used since the 1920s for this very purpose. it had been researchers and physicians at Johns Hopkins center who observed that these diets, in patients with epilepsy, helped reduce disorders like seizures.

Since the sixties, these diets are widely used for the treatment of obesity, but also within the presence of other pathological conditions like diabetes, polycystic ovary syndrome, acne, it had been observed that additionally to working on convulsions, produced positive effects on the body fat, blood glucose, cholesterol, and hunger levels.

The ketogenic diet has, therefore, increasingly established itself as a diet to reduce, which exploits the results for the body of the reduction of carbohydrates and therefore the increased consumption of fats not for therapeutic purposes but to stimulate weight loss.

There is not just one sort of ketogenic diet. Ketogenic diets are all highly hyperlipidemic diets, which include a robust reduction within the intake of carbohydrates (on average, no quite 50 g per day) and therefore the intake of protein sources mainly of high biological value. Among these, the Atkins diet, the Blackburn diet, the Tisanoreica diet, the primary phases of the Dukan Diet.

Ketogenic diet to lose weight: the principles

The ketogenic diet is predicated on a robust reduction within the consumption of carbohydrates, related to a considerable increase within the consumption of fats and a high intake of proteins.

It, therefore, determines a considerable imbalance, almost a reversal, of the proportions between the macronutrients provided by the Mediterranean diet, which recommends an intake of carbohydrates adequate to 45-60% of daily energy, fats adequate to no quite 35%, and proteins adequate to 10-12%.

In the ketogenic diet, on the opposite hand, fats represent 70-75% of the entire calories ingested, carbohydrates don't exceed 5-10% and proteins are around 15-25% of the daily calorie intake.

Unlike other low-carb diets, the keto diet doesn't, therefore, include an excessive load of proteins, which are present during a greater measure than within the Mediterranean diet, but whose increase isn't as drastic as that of fats.

Types of the ketogenic diet

Although the essential principles remain an equivalent (reduction of carbohydrates, a robust increase in fats, consistent presence of proteins), there's not only one ketogenic diet but there are often different variations of it, with different proportions of the varied nutrients, a cyclic increase within the intake of carbohydrates, caloric restrictions and specific formulas for vegetarians and vegans.

The main variants of the ketogenic diet

Standard Ketogenic Diet (SKD): this is often the foremost classic and the strictest keto diet, which consists of obtaining about 75% of calories from fat, 5% from carbohydrates, and 20% from proteins.

Modified Ketogenic Diet (MKD): also this program foresees a discount within the intake of carbohydrates, but less drastic, that's adequate to 30% of the daily caloric intake. Fats and proteins cover, respectively, 40% and 30% of the entire daily calories.

Cyclical Ketogenic Diet (CKD): this is often a variant of the ketogenic diet that gives for a rise within the intake of carbohydrates (technically we mention "recharge") during a cyclic way, usually 1-2 times every week. it's designed for those that have difficulty sticking to a diet with such low carbohydrate content, especially a day and for extended periods.

Targeted Ketogenic Diet (TKD): this diet plan is meant for those that do sports and allows you to feature carbohydrates on training days.

High Protein Keto Diet (HPKD): this version of the keto diet is usually followed by those that want to preserve muscle mass, like bodybuilders or the elderly. The protein share is 30%, the fat share is 65%, carbohydrates are reduced, as within the classic ketogenic diet, to 5%.

Keto vegan or vegetarian diet: these variants of the ketogenic diet replace animal-based foods with plant-based foods, like nuts, seeds, fruits, and vegetables low in carbohydrates, healthy fats, and fermented foods.

Dirty Keto Diet: during this variant of the ketogenic diet, the proportions between the nutrients are equivalent because the classic one, but rather than healthy fats, unhealthy fats are consumed, with concessions even to sodas and nutriment.

The lazy ketogenic diet (Lazy Keto): this version is defined as "lazy" because it provides only a strict calculation of carbohydrates taken daily, which must not exceed 20 g, while it leaves the intake of fats and proteins not precisely monitored.

Keto diet: why does it cause you to lose weight?

The ketogenic diet is predicated on the idea that if we take a high amount of carbohydrates and thus sugars, these are going to be stored within the body within the sort of body fat, resulting in weight gain.

If the intake of carbohydrates is strongly reduced, the body, which usually uses them as its primary source of energy, are going to be forced to use instead fats, both the stored ones and people introduced through food.

This causes the body to rapidly reduce and burn fat, while continuing to require calories in amounts capable of its needs and, indeed, without the necessity to count them and without feeling hungry.

The imbalance between nutrients, therefore, aims to switch the body's energy metabolism, causing it to use fats rather than carbohydrates as fuel, to supply weight loss.

Ketosis

But what happens to the body if it stops taking in most carbohydrates? The intake of either a really low proportion of carbohydrates or a high proportion of fats triggers a state of ketosis.

Ketosis may be a metabolic condition during which the body is induced to supply so-called "ketone bodies", which it'll use as an energy source rather than sugars.

How do I enter a state of ketosis?

Ketosis is often reached after a couple of days of total fasting, which, however, wouldn't be sustainable for the body: the ketogenic diet "tricks" the body, depriving it of carbohydrates, to induce it to act as after a quick, that's to use fats as an energy source, thus losing weight.

But how is it possible to succeed in the state of ketosis?

you must reduce the intake of glucose from the consumption of foods containing carbohydrates (cereals, but also vegetables that are rich in them);
the reduction of carbohydrates forces the body to seek out an alternate source of energy, namely fats;
in the absence of glucose, the body begins to burn fat and produces ketones;
when the ketones within the blood reach a particular level, you enter a state of ketosis that causes weight loss.

Ketogenic diet: what to eat

The three basic rules to realize the state of ketosis is:
habitually eat foods without carbohydrates
limit foods that provide moderate amounts
avoid foods rich in carbohydrates.
Here are, in detail, the recommended foods (to be consumed regularly or occasionally, consistent with their content of carbohydrates) and people not recommended, which should be avoided.

Recommended foods, to be consumed regularly

Fats
The fats considered healthy by the ketogenic diet are saturated fats, monounsaturated fats, and certain sorts of polyunsaturated fats (PUFA), particularly omega-3 fatty acids. the recommendation is to incorporate all kinds of fats in your daily diet, with a greater emphasis on saturated fats.
These include vegetable oil, copra oil, butter, palm oil, avocado oil, lard, flaxseed.

Protein
According to the keto diet, protein sources richer in fats are to be preferred.
Among these, red and red meat (beef, lamb, veal, liver, chicken, turkey, quail, goose, duck), eggs, fish (tuna, trout, anchovy, salmon, sardine, mackerel, plaice).

Vegetables
All non-starchy vegetables that contain very low proportions of carbohydrates are allowed.
These include green leafy vegetables like Swiss chard, arugula, chicory, radicchio, fennel, spinach, cruciferous vegetables (broccoli, cabbage, and cauliflower), celery, cucumbers, zucchini, chives, and leeks.

Tomatoes, asparagus, mushrooms, peppers, green beans, bamboo shoots, and soybeans contain higher but acceptable, amounts of carbohydrates so that they are often routinely included during a ketogenic diet.

Fruits
Fatty fruits like avocados are often consumed on the ketogenic diet.

Condiments
Spices and herbs, apple vinegar, unsweetened mustard.

Drinks
Water, coffee, and tea without sugar (in moderation).

In this book, there are several recipes for a keto diet and you'll choose the varied dishes for your daily diet trying to urge the proper calories you would like. Enjoy!

Breakfast

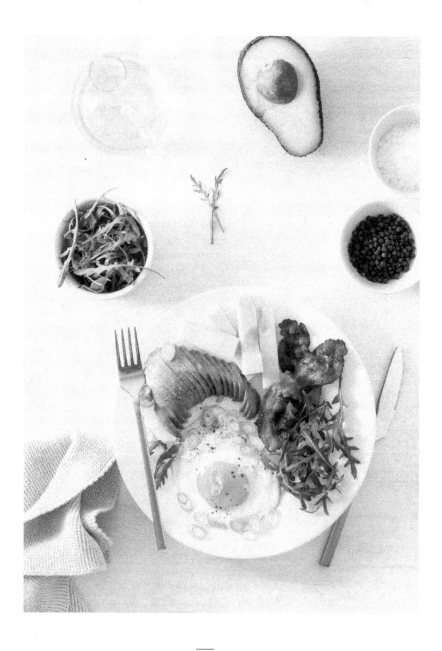

Cheesy Broccoli Muffins

Preparation Time: 15 minutes
Cooking Time: 20 minutes
Servings: 6

Ingredients:
2 tablespoons unsalted butter
6 large organic eggs
1/2 cup heavy whipping cream
1/2 cup Parmesan cheese, grated
Salt and ground black pepper, as required
11/4 cups broccoli, chopped
2 tablespoons fresh parsley, chopped
1/2 cup Swiss cheese, grated

Directions:
Grease a 12-cup muffin tin. In a bowl or container, put in the cream, eggs, Parmesan cheese, salt, and black pepper, and beat until well combined. Divide the broccoli and parsley in the bottom of each prepared muffin cup evenly. Top with the egg mixture, followed by the Swiss cheese. Let the muffins bake for about 20 minutes, rotating the pan once halfway through. Carefully, invert the muffins onto a serving platter and serve warm.

Nutrition:
Calories 241 | Fat 11.5g | Fiber 8.5g
Carbohydrates 4.1 g | Protein: 11.1g

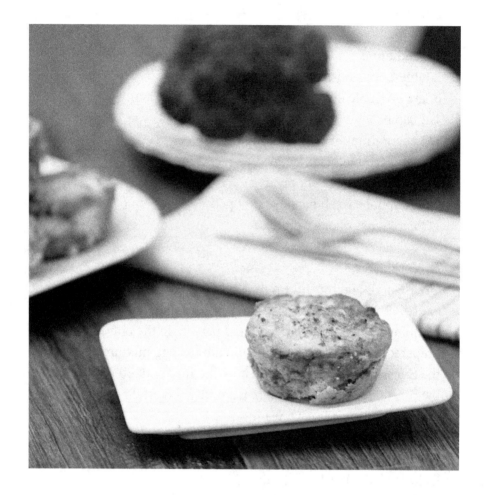

Peanut Butter Oatmeal

Preparation time: 10 minutes
Cooking time: 8 hours
Servings: 2

Ingredients:
1 banana, mashed
and ½ cups almond milk
½ cup steel cut oats
tablespoons peanut butter
½ teaspoon vanilla extract
½ teaspoon cinnamon powder ½ tablespoon chia seeds

Directions:
In your slow cooker, mix almond milk with banana, oats, peanut butter, vanilla extract, cinnamon and chia, stir, cover and cook on Low for 8 hours.
Stir oatmeal one more time, divide into 2 bowls and serve.
Enjoy!

Nutrition:
Calories 222 | Fat 5 | Fiber 6 | Carbs 9 | Protein 11

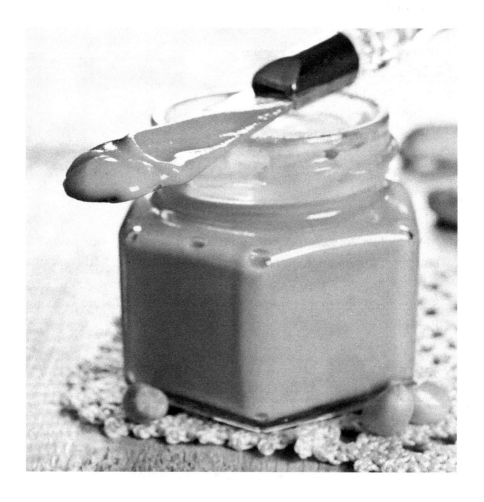

Vanilla Pumpkin Bread

Preparation time: 10 minutes
Cooking time: 2 hours
Servings: 2

Ingredients:
Cooking spray
½ cup white flour
½ cup whole wheat flour
½ teaspoon baking soda
pinch of cinnamon powder
2 tablespoons olive oil
2 tablespoons maple syrup
egg
½ tablespoon milk
½ teaspoon vanilla extract
½ cup pumpkin puree
tablespoons walnuts, chopped
2 tablespoons chocolate chips

Directions:
In a bowl, mix white flour with whole wheat flour, baking soda and cinnamon and stir. Add maple syrup, olive oil, egg, milk, vanilla extract, pumpkin puree, walnuts and chocolate chips and stir well. Grease a loaf pan that fits your slow cooker with cooking spray, pour pumpkin bread, transfer to your cooker and cook on High for 2 hours. Slice bread, divide between plates and serve.
Enjoy!

Nutrition:
calories 200 | fat 3 | fiber 5 | Carbs 8 |Protein 4

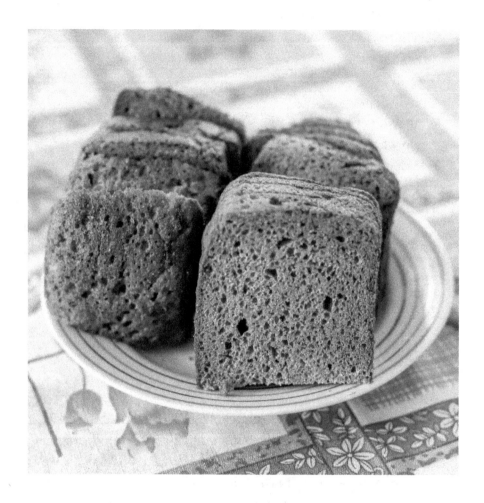

Sweet potato breakfast pie

Preparation time: 10 minutes
Cooking time: 7 hours
Servings: 6

Ingredients:
1 shredded sweet potato (peeled)
1 pound turkey bacon
9 eggs
1 small diced sweet onion
1 tsp. cinnamon
1 tsp. dried basil
Salt and pepper

Directions:
Grease your slow cooker as you would a baking dish.
Shred the sweet potato and get all ingredients ready.
Cut the bacon into small pieces.
Then whisk the eggs and add all the ingredients into the slow cooker.
Cook on low temperature for 7 to 8 hours.
You can serve it as a pie, by cutting slices or like a cake cutting squares.

Nutrition:
245 Cal | 11.5 g total fat (4.6 g sat. fat) | 152 mg chop |
189 mg sodium !7.5 g carb | 3.9g fiber | 9.6. G protein.

Rosemary Turkey Sausage Egg Muffins

Preparation time: 5 minutes
Cooking time: 15 minutes
Servings: 3

Ingredient:
1 teaspoon butter
6 eggs
Salt and black pepper, to taste
½ teaspoon dried rosemary
1 cup pecorino romano cheese, grated
3 turkey sausages, chopped

Directions:
Preheat oven to 400°F (205°C) and grease muffin cups with cooking spray.
In a skillet over medium heat add the butter and cook the turkey sausages for 4-5 minutes.
Beat 3 eggs with a fork. Add in sausages, cheese, and seasonings.
Divide between the muffin cups and bake for 4 minutes. Crack in an egg to each of the cups. Bake for an additional 4 minutes. Allow cooling before serving.

Nutritions:
calories: 422 | fat: 34.2g | protein: 26.4g | carbs: 2.1g | net carbs: 2.1g | fiber: 0g

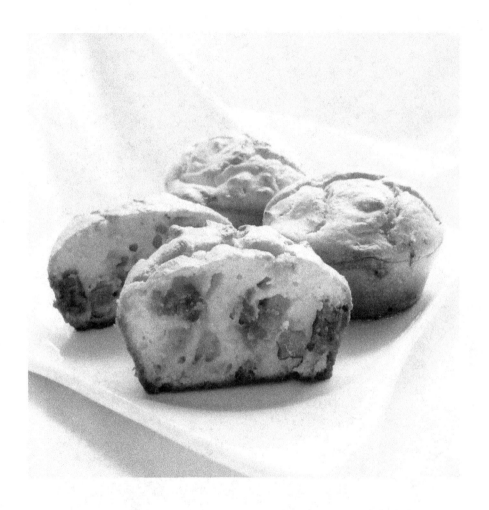

Chicken

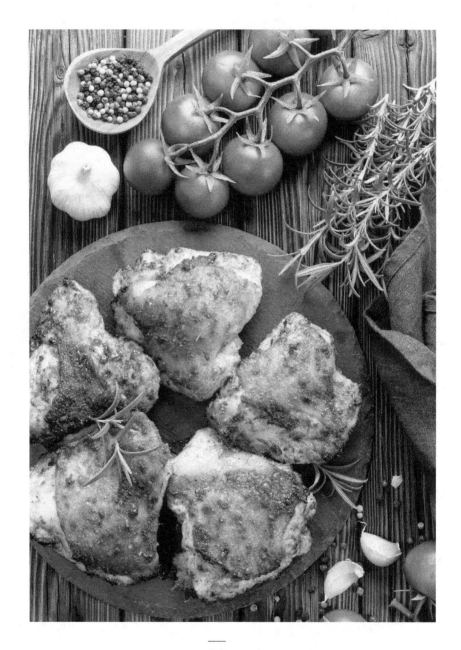

Olla Tapada

Preparation time: 15 minutes
Cooking time: 25 minutes
Servings: 3

Ingrediens:
2 teaspoons canola oil
1 red bell pepper, deveined and chopped
1 shallot, chopped
½ cup celery rib, chopped
½ cup chayote, peeled and cubed
1 pound (454 g) duck breasts, boneless, skinless, and chopped into small chunks
1½ cups vegetable broth
½ stick Mexican cinnamon
1 thyme sprig
1 rosemary sprig

Directions:
Sea salt and freshly ground black pepper, to taste
Heat the canola oil in a soup pot (or clay pot) over a medium-high flame. Now, sauté the bell pepper, shallot and celery until they have softened about 5 minutes.
Add the remaining ingredients and stir to combine. Once it starts boiling, turn the heat to simmer and partially cover the pot.
Let it simmer for 17 to 20 minutes or until thoroughly cooked. Enjoy!

Nutritions:
calories: 230 | fat: 9.6g | protein: 30.5g | carbs: 3.3g | net carbs: 2.3g | fiber: 1.

Cheesy Bacon Ranch Chicken

Preparation Time: 40 minutes
Cooking Time: 35 minutes
Servings: 8

Ingredients:
8 boneless and skinned chicken breasts
1 cup of olive oil
8 thick slices bacon
3 cups of shredded mozzarella
1 1/4 tablespoon of ranch seasoning
1 small chopped onion
Chopped chives
Kosher salt or pink salt
Black pepper

Directions:
Preheat skillet and heat little oil, and cook bacon evenly on both sides. Save four tablespoons of drippings and put the others away. Add in salt and pepper in a bowl and rub it over chicken to season. Put 1/2 oil on the flame to cook the chicken from each side for 5 to 7 minutes. When ready, reduce the heat and put in the ranch seasoning, then add mozzarella. Cover and cook on a low flame for 3-5 minutes. Put in bacon fat and chopped chives, then bacon and cover it. Take off and serve warm.

Nutrition:
Calories 387 | Fat 15.1g | Fiber 10.6g |
Carbohydrates 5.9 g | Protein 12.9g

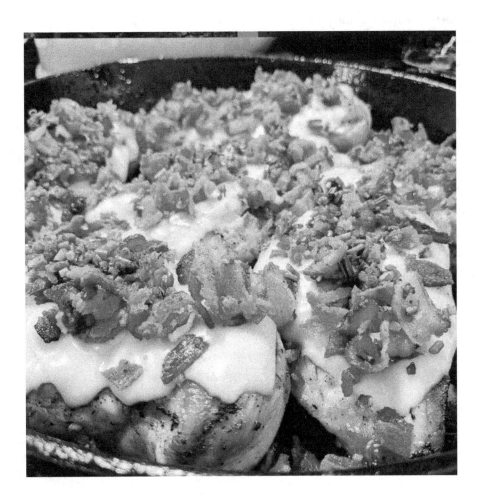

Pepper, Cheese, and Sauerkraut Stuffed Chicken

Preparation time: 15 minutes
Cooking time: 30 minutes
Servings: 5
Ingredients:
2 tablespoons olive oil
5 chicken cutlets
½ teaspoon cayenne pepper
½ teaspoon oregano
Sea salt and ground black pepper, to taste
tablespoon Dijon mustard
garlic cloves, minced
5 Italian peppers, deveined and chopped
1 chili pepper, chopped
1 cup Romano cheese, shredded
5 tablespoons sauerkraut, for serving

Directions:

Brush a baking pan with 1 tablespoon of the olive oil. Bruch the chicken cutlets with the remaining tablespoon of olive oil.

Season the chicken cutlets with the cayenne pepper, oregano, salt, and black pepper. Spread mustard on one side of each chicken cutlet. Divide the garlic, peppers, and Romano cheese on the mustard side. Roll up tightly and use toothpicks to secure your rolls. Transfer to the prepared baking pan.

Bake in the preheated oven at 370°F (188°C) for about 30 minutes until golden brown on all sides (an instant-read thermometer should register 165°F (74°C)).

Spoon the sauerkraut over the chicken and serve. Bon appétit!

376 Calories; 16.7g Fat; 5.8g Carbs; 47g Protein; 1g Fiber

Nutrition:

calories 378 | fat 16.6g | protein 47.0g | carbs 5.7g | net carbs 4.7g | fiber 1.0g

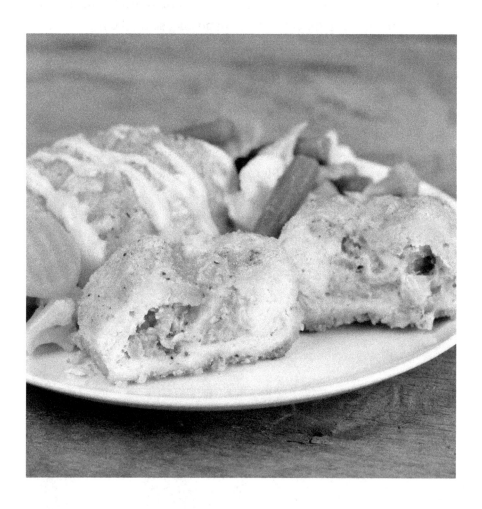

Mediterranean Roasted Chicken Drumettes

Preparation time: 15 minutes
Cooking time: 20 minutes
Servings: 5
 Ingredients:
2 tablespoons olive oil
1½ pounds (680 g) chicken drumettes
2 cloves garlic, minced
1 thyme sprig
rosemary sprig
½ teaspoon dried oregano
Sea salt and freshly ground black pepper, to taste
tablespoons Greek cooking wine
½ cup chicken bone broth
red onion, cut into wedges
bell peppers, sliced
Directions:
Start by preheating your oven to 420ºF (216ºC). Brush the sides and bottom a baking dish with 1 tablespoon of olive oil.
Heat the remaining tablespoon of olive oil in a saucepan over a moderate flame. Brown the chicken drumettes for 5 to 6 minutes per side.
Transfer the warm chicken drumettes to a baking dish. Add the garlic, spices, wine and broth. Scatter red onion and peppers around chicken drumettes.
Roast in the preheated oven for about 13 minutes. Serve immediately and enjoy!
Nutrition:
calories 219 | fat 9.2g | protein 28.5g | carbs 4.2g | net carbs 3.5g | fiber 0.7g

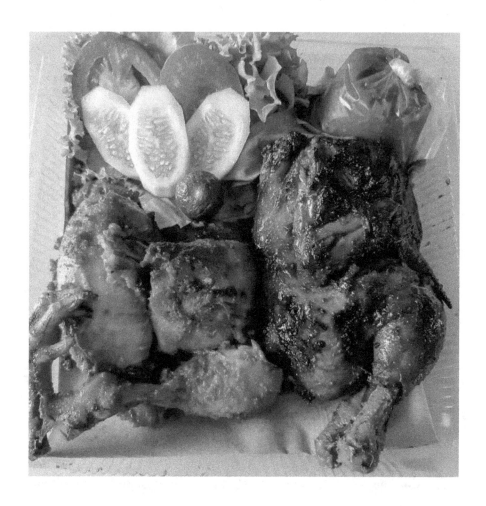

Chimichurri Chicken Tender

Preparation time: 10 minutes
Cooking time: 35 minutes
Servings: 5

Ingredients:
½ cup fresh parsley, chopped
¼ cup olive oil
4 tablespoons white wine vinegar
2 garlic cloves, minced
1½ pounds (680 g) chicken tenders
Sea salt and ground black pepper, to taste
1 cup sour cream

Directions:
In a food processor or blender, process the parsley, olive oil, vinegar, and garlic until chunky sauce forms. Now, pierce the chicken randomly with a small knife.
Pour half of the chimichurri sauce on top, cover, and refrigerate for 1 hour; discard the chimichurri sauce.
Brush the sides and bottom of a baking pan with nonstick cooking spray. Arrange the chicken tenders in the baking pan.
Then, season your chicken with salt and black pepper to taste. Pour in the sour cream and bake in the preheated oven at 370°F (188°C) for 35 minutes or until cooked through.
Serve with the remaining chimichurri sauce. Bon appétit!

Nutrition:
calories 316 | fat: 29.8g | protein 29.4g | carbs 4.0g | net carbs 3.8g | fiber 0.

Pork

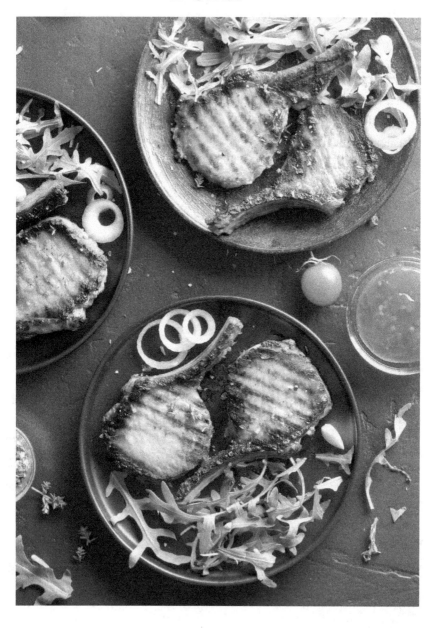

Shepherd's Pie

Preparation Time: 5 minutes
Cooking Time: 3-9 minutes
Servings: 2

Ingredients:
1/4 cup olive oil
1-pound grass-fed ground beef
1/2 cup celery, chopped
1/4 cup yellow onion, chopped
3 garlic cloves, minced
cup tomatoes, chopped
(12-ounce) packages riced cauliflower, cooked and well-drained
1 cup cheddar cheese, shredded
1/4 cup Parmesan cheese, shredded
1 cup heavy cream 1 teaspoon dried thyme

Directions:
Preheat your oven to 350°F.
Heat oil heat and cook the ground beef, celery, onions, and garlic for about 8–10 minutes. Immediately stir in the tomatoes. Transfer mixture into a 10x7-inch casserole dish evenly. In a food processor, add the cauliflower, cheeses, cream, thyme, and pulse until a mashed potatoes-like mixture is formed. Spread the cauliflower mixture over the meat in the casserole dish evenly. Bake for about 35–40 minutes. Cut into desired sized pieces and serve.

Nutrition:
Calories 387 | Fat 11.5g | Fiber 9.4g ! Carbohydrates 5.5 g | Protein 18.5g

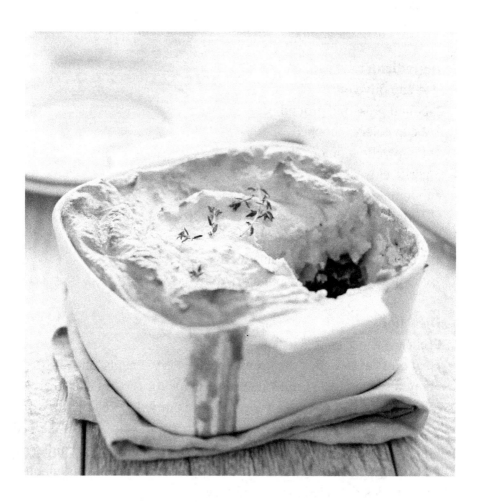

Pork, Squash, and Mushroom Casserole

Preparation time: 15 minutes
Cooking time: 30 minutes
Servings: 4

Ingredients:
1 pound (454 g) ground pork
1 large yellow squash, thinly sliced
Salt and black pepper to taste
1 clove garlic, minced
4 green onions, chopped
1 cup chopped cremini mushrooms
1 (15-ounce / 425-g) can diced tomatoes
½ cup pork rinds, crushed
¼ cup chopped parsley
1 cup cottage cheese
1 cup Mexican cheese blend
3 tablespoons olive oil
⅓ cup water

Directions:

Preheat the oven to 370°F (188°C).

Heat the olive oil in a skillet over medium heat, add the pork, season it with salt and black pepper, and cook for 3 minutes or until no longer pink. Stir occasionally while breaking any lumps apart. Add the garlic, half of the green onions, mushrooms, and 2 tablespoons of pork rinds. Cook for 3 minutes. Stir in the tomatoes, half of the parsley, and water. Cook further for 3 minutes, and then turn the heat off. Mix the remaining parsley, cottage cheese, and Mexican cheese blend. Set aside. Sprinkle the bottom of a baking dish with 3 tablespoons of pork rinds; top with half of the squash and a season of salt, ⅔ of the pork mixture, and the cheese mixture. Repeat the layering process a second time to exhaust the ingredients. Cover the baking dish with foil and bake for 20 minutes. After, remove the foil and brown the top of the casserole with the broiler side of the oven for 2 minutes. Remove the dish when ready and serve warm.

Nutrition:

calories 496 | fat 29.1g | protein 36.6g | carbs 7.1g | net carbs 2.6g | fiber 4.5g

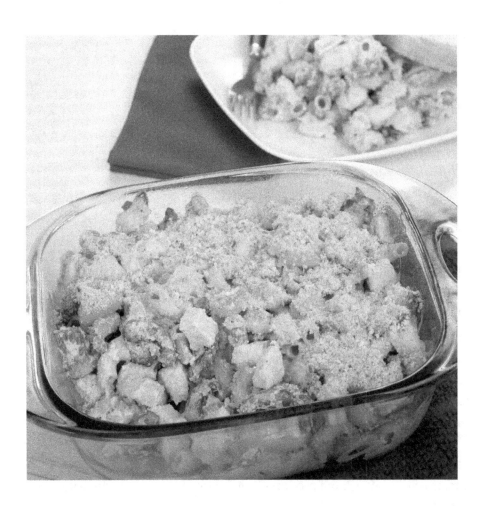

White Wine Pork with Cabbage

Preparation time: 15 minutes
Cooking time: 1 hour 15 minutes
Servings: 6

Ingredients:
2 tablespoons olive oil
2 pounds (907 g) pork stew meat, cubed
Salt and black pepper, to taste
2 tablespoons butter
4 garlic cloves, minced
¾ cup vegetable stock
½ cup white wine
3 carrots, chopped
1 cabbage head, shredded
½ cup scallions, chopped
1 cup heavy cream

Directions:
Set a pan over medium heat and warm butter and oil. Sear the pork until brown. Add garlic, scallions and carrots; sauté for 5 minutes. Pour in the cabbage, stock and wine, and bring to a boil. Reduce the heat and cook for 1 hour covered. Add in heavy cream as you stir for 1 minute, adjust seasonings and serve.

Nutrition:
calories 512 | fat: 32.6g | protein 42.9g | carbs 9.3g | net carbs 5.9g | fiber 3.4g

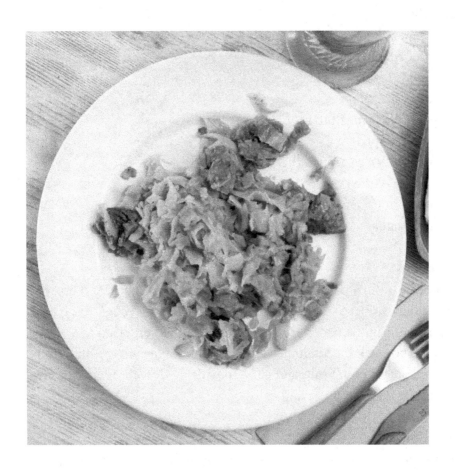

Pork and Cauliflower Goulash

Preparation time: 15 minutes
Cooking time: 10 minutes
Servings: 4

Ingredients:
red bell pepper, seeded and chopped
tablespoons olive oil
1½ pounds (680 g) ground pork
Salt and black pepper, to taste
2 cups cauliflower florets
1 onion, chopped
14 ounces (397 g) canned diced tomatoes
¼ teaspoon garlic powder
1 tablespoon tomato purée
1½ cups water

Directions:
Heat olive oil in a pan over medium heat, stir in the pork, and brown for 5 minutes. Place in the bell pepper and onion, and cook for 4 minutes. Stir in the water, tomatoes, and cauliflower, bring to a simmer and cook for 5 minutes while covered. Place in the black pepper, tomato paste, salt, and garlic powder. Stir well, remove from the heat, split into bowls, and enjoy.

Nutrition:
calories 476 | fat 36.9g | protein 43.9g | carbs 8.3g | net carbs 4.4g | fiber 3.9g

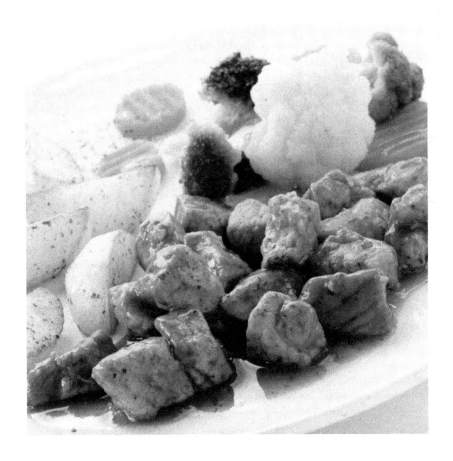

Herbed Pork and Turkey Meatloaf

Preparation time: 20 minutes
Cooking time: 60 minutes
Servings: 6

Ingredients:
pound (454 g)ground pork
½ pound (227 g) ground turkey
¼ cup flax seed meal
eggs, beaten
2 cloves garlic, minced
½ cup scallions, chopped
Sea salt and ground black pepper, to season
1 teaspoon dried oregano
½ teaspoon dried basil
½ teaspoon dried marjoram
½ teaspoon dried rosemary
1 tablespoon fresh chives, chopped
3 ounces (85 g) tomato paste
1 tablespoon coconut aminos
1 tablespoon brown mustard

Directions:

Begin by preheating your oven to 360°F (182°C). Now, spritz the sides and bottom of a loaf pan with nonstick cooking oil.

Thoroughly combine the ground meat with the flax seed meal, eggs, garlic, scallions, spices, and herbs.

Press the mixture into the prepared loaf pan. Bake in the preheated oven for 30 minutes

In a mixing bowl, whisk the tomato paste, coconut aminos, and mustard. Spread the mixture on top of the meatloaf.

Return to the oven; bake for a further 30 minutes or until internal temperature reaches 165°F (74°C). Bon appétit!

Nutrition:

Calories 345 | fat 23.2g | protein 30.1g | carbs 2.7g | net carbs 1.7g | fiber 1.0g

Beef and Lamb

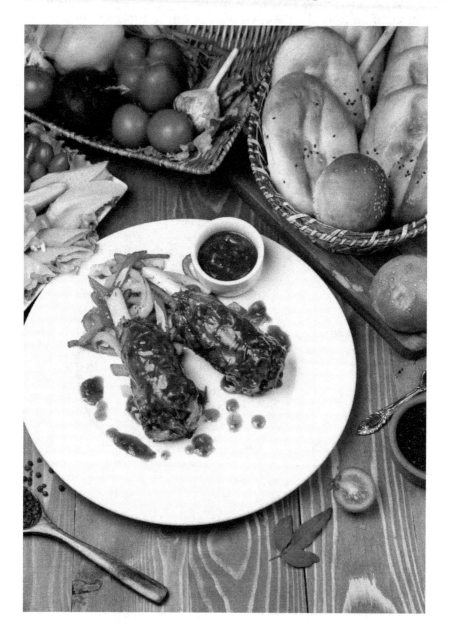

Beef and Broccoli Casserole

Preparation time: 15 minutes
Cooking time: 4 hours
Servings: 6

Ingredients:
tablespoon olive oil
pounds (907 g) ground beef
head broccoli, cut into florets
Salt and black pepper, to taste
teaspoons mustard
2 teaspoons Worcestershire sauce
28 ounces (794 g) canned diced tomatoes
2 cups Mozzarella cheese, grated
16 ounces (454 g) tomato sauce
2 tablespoons fresh parsley, chopped
1 teaspoon dried oregano

Directions:
Apply black pepper and salt to the broccoli florets, set them into a bowl, drizzle over the olive oil, and toss well to coat completely. In a separate bowl, combine the beef with Worcestershire sauce, salt, mustard, and black pepper, and stir well. Press on the slow cooker's bottom. Scatter in the broccoli, add the tomatoes, parsley, Mozzarella, oregano, and tomato sauce. Cook for 4 hours on low; covered. Split the casserole among bowls and enjoy while hot.

Nutrition:
calories 435 | fat 21.1g | protein 50.9g | carbs 13.5g | net carbs 5.5g | fiber 8.0g

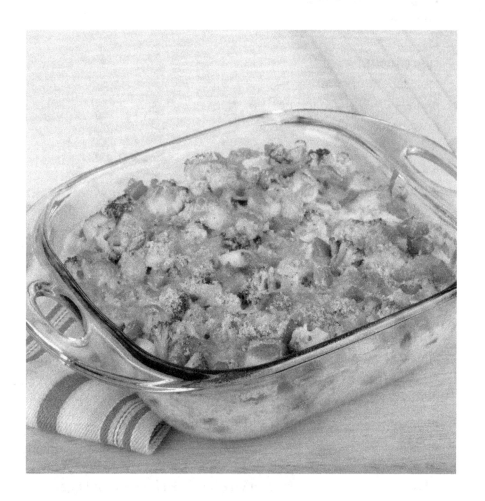

Pork Rind Crusted Beef Meatballs

Preparation time: 10 minutes
Cooking time: 40 minutes
Servings: 5

Ingredients:
½ cup pork rinds, crushed
1 egg
Salt and black pepper, to taste
1½ pounds (680 g) ground beef
10 ounces (283 g) canned onion soup
1 tablespoon almond flour
¼ cup free-sugar ketchup
3 teaspoons Worcestershire sauce
½ teaspoon dry mustard
¼ cup water

Directions:
In a bowl, combine ⅓ cup of the onion soup with the beef, pepper, pork rinds, egg, and salt. Heat a pan over medium heat, shape the mixture into 12 meatballs. Brown in the pan for 12 minutes on both sides.
In a separate bowl, combine the rest of the soup with the almond flour, dry mustard, ketchup, Worcestershire sauce, and water. Pour this over the beef meatballs, cover the pan, and cook for 20 minutes as you stir occasionally. Split among serving bowls and serve.

Nutrition:
Calories 333 | fat 18.1g | protein 24.9g | carbs 7.4g | net carbs 6.9g | fiber 0.5g

Beef Chuck Roast with Mushrooms

Preparation time: 15 minutes
Cooking time: 3 hours 10 minutes
Servings: 6

Ingredients:
2 pounds (907 g) beef chuck roast, cubed
2 tablespoons olive oil
14.5 ounces (411 g) canned diced tomatoes
2 carrots, chopped
Salt and black pepper, to taste
½ pound (227 g) mushrooms, sliced
2 celery stalks, chopped
2 yellow onions, chopped
1 cup beef stock
1 tablespoon fresh thyme, chopped
½ teaspoon dry mustard
3 tablespoons almond flour

Directions:
Set an ovenproof pot over medium heat, warm olive oil and brown
the beef on each side for a few minutes. Stir in the tomatoes, onions,
salt, pepper, mustard, carrots, mushrooms, celery, and stock.
In a bowl, combine 1 cup water with flour. Place this to the pot, stir
then set in the oven, and bake for 3 hours at 325°F (163°C) stirring at
intervals of 30 minutes. Scatter the fresh thyme over and serve
warm.

Nutrition:
calories 326 | fat 18.1g | protein 28.1g | carbs 10.4g | net carbs 6.9g |
fiber 3.5g

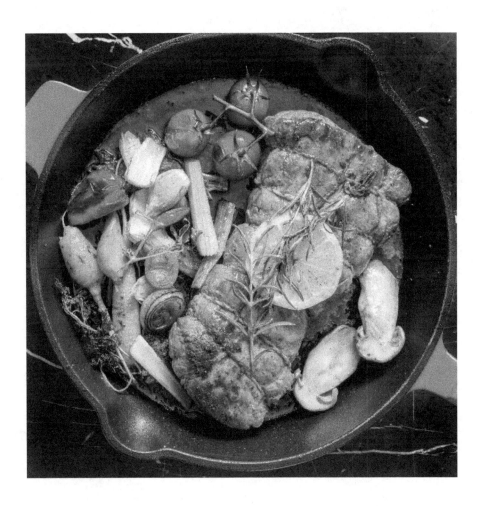

Parmesan Beef Meatball alla Parmigiana

Preparation time: 10 minutes
Cooking time: 40 minutes
Servings: 4

Ingredients:
For the Meatballs
 pound (454 g) ground beef (80/20)
tablespoons chopped fresh parsley, plus more for garnish if desired
⅓ cup grated Parmesan cheese
¼ cup superfine blanched almond flour
1 large egg, beaten
1 teaspoon kosher salt
¼ teaspoon ground black pepper
¼ teaspoon garlic powder ¼ teaspoon onion powder
¼ teaspoon dried oregano leaves
¼ cup warm filtered water
1 cup marinara sauce, store-bought or homemade
1 cup shredded whole-milk Mozzarella cheese

Directions:

Preheat the oven to 350°F (180°C). Line a 15 by 10-inch sheet pan with foil or parchment paper. Put the ground beef, parsley, Parmesan, almond flour, egg, salt, pepper, garlic powder, onion powder, oregano, and water in a medium-sized bowl. Mix thoroughly by hand until fully combined. Form the meat mixture into 12 meatballs about 2 inches in diameter and place them 2 inches apart on the sheet pan. Bake for 20 minutes. Place the meatballs in a casserole dish large enough to fit all of the meatballs. Spoon the marinara evenly over the meatballs, then sprinkle the cheese over the meatballs. Bake for 20 minutes, or until the meatballs are cooked through, the sauce is bubbling, and the cheese is golden. Garnish with chopped fresh parsley, if desired.

Nutrition:

calories 431 | fat 30.9g | protein 32.9g | carbs 4.8g | net carbs 2.8g | fiber 2.0g

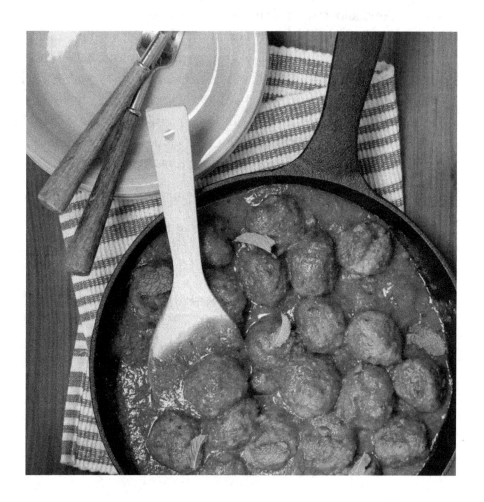

Simple Pesto Beef Chuck Roast

Preparating time: 5 minutes
Cooking time: 9 to 10 hours
Servings: 8

Ingredients:
1 tablespoon extra-virgin olive oil 2 pounds (907 g) beef chuck roast
¾ cup prepared pesto
½ cup beef broth

Directions:
Lightly grease the insert of the slow cooker with the olive oil.
Slather the pesto all over the beef. Place the beef in the insert and pour in the broth.
Cover and cook on low for 9 to 10 hours.
Serve warm.

Nutrition:
calories 529 | fat 42.9g | protein 31.9g | carbs 1.9g | net carbs 1.9g | fiber 0g

Fish and Seafood

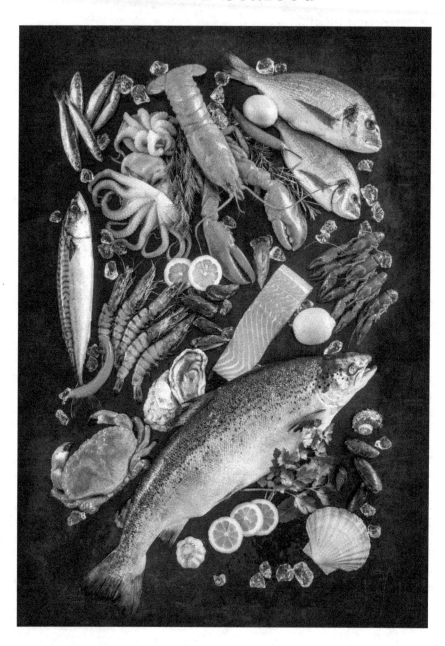

Tuna Cakes

Preparation Time: 15 minutes
Cooking Time: 10 minutes
Servings: 2

Ingredients:
 (15-ounce) can water-packed tuna, drained
1/2 celery stalk, chopped
tablespoon fresh parsley, chopped
teaspoon fresh dill, chopped
tablespoons walnuts, chopped
2 tablespoons mayonnaise
1 organic egg, beaten
1 tablespoon butter
3 cups lettuce

Directions:
For burgers: Add all ingredients (except the butter and lettuce) in a bowl and mix until well combined.
Make two equal-sized patties from the mixture.
Melt some butter and cook the patties for about 2–3 minutes.
Carefully flip the side and cook for about 2–3 minutes.
Divide the lettuce onto serving plates.
Top each plate with one burger and serve.

Nutrition:
Calories: 267 | Fat: 12.5g | Fiber: 9.4g | Carbohydrates:3.8 g | Protein: 11.5g

Lemon Scallops

Preparation time: 10 minutes
Cooking time: 1 hours
Servings: 4

Ingredients:
1-pound scallops
1 teaspoon salt
1 teaspoon ground white pepper
½ teaspoon olive oil
3 tablespoons lemon juice
1 teaspoon lemon zest, grated
1 tablespoon dried oregano
½ cup of water

Directions
Sprinkle the scallops with salt, ground white pepper, lemon juice, and lemon zest and leave for 10-15 minutes to marinate.
After this, sprinkle the scallops with olive oil and dried oregano.
Put the scallops in the slow cooker and add water.
Cook the seafood on High for 1 hour.

Nutrition:
113 calories | 19.3g protein | 4.1g carbohydrates | 1.7g fat |
0.7g fiber | 37mg cholesterol | 768mg sodium | 407mg potassium

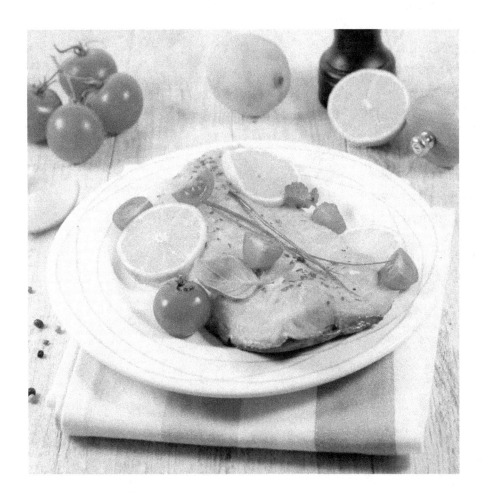

Pan-Seared Cod with Tomato Hollandaise

Preparation Time: 10 minutes
Cooking Time: 10 minutes
Servings: 4

Ingredients:
 Pan-Seared Cod
1 pound (4-fillets) wild Alaskan Cod
1 tbsp. salted butter
1 tbsp. olive oil
Tomato Hollandaise
3 large egg yolks
3 tbsp. warm water
226 grams salted butter, melted
1/4 tsp. salt
1/4 tsp. black pepper
2 tbsp. tomato paste 2 tbsp. fresh lemon juice

Directions:

Season both sides of the code fillet without salt, the salt will be added in the last. Heat a skillet over medium heat and coat with olive oil and butter. When the butter heats up, place the cod fillet in the skillet and sear on both sides for 2-3 minutes. Baste the fish fillet with the oil and butter mixture. You will know that the cod cooked when it easily flakes when poked with a fork. Melt the butter in the microwave. In a double boil, beat egg yolks with warm water until thick and creamy and start forming soft peaks. Remove the double boil from the heat, gradually adding the melted butter and stirring. Season. Mix in the tomato paste. Stir to combine. Pour in the water and lemon juice to lighten the sauce texture.

Nutrition:

Calories: 356 | Fat: 16.1g | Fiber: 12.3g | Carbohydrates:3.1 g Protein: 18.4g

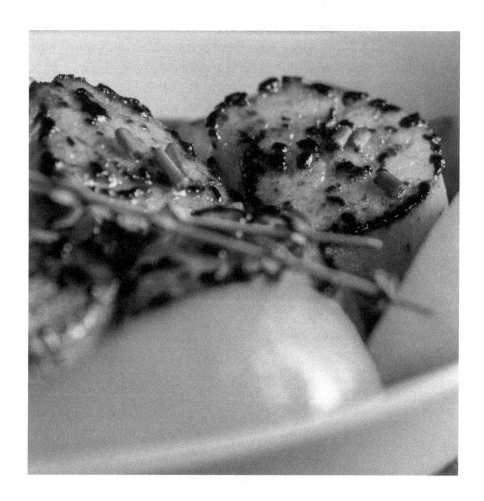

Garlic-Lemon Mahi Mahi

Preparation Time: 15 minutes
Cooking Time: 10 minutes
Servings: 3

Ingredients:
6 tablespoons of butter
5 tablespoons of extra-virgin olive oil
4 ounces of mahi-mahi fillets
3 minced cloves of garlic
Kosher salt
Black pepper
2 pounds of asparagus
2 sliced lemons
Zest and juice of 2 lemons
1 teaspoon of crushed red pepper flakes
1 tablespoon of chopped parsley

Directions:
Melt three tablespoons of butter and olive oil in a microwave.
Heat a skillet and put in mahi-mahi, then sprinkle black pepper.
For around 5 minutes per side, cook it. When done, move to a plate.
In another skillet, add remaining oil and add in the asparagus, stir fry
for 2-3 minutes. Take out on a plate.
In the same skillet, pour in the remaining butter, and add garlic, red
pepper, lemon, zest, juice, and parsley.
Add in the mahi-mahi and asparagus and stir together. Serve hot.

Nutrition:
Calories: 317 | Fat: 8.5g | Fiber: 6.9g | Carbohydrates:3.1 g |
Protein: 16.1g

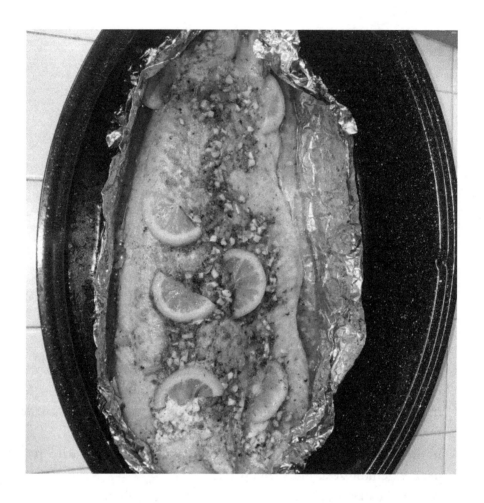

Dijon Crab Cakes

Preparation time: 10 minutes
Cooking time: 5 minutes
Servings: 4

Ingredients:
1 tablespoon coconut oil
1 pound (454 g) lump crab meat
1 teaspoon Dijon mustard
1 egg
¼ cup mayonnaise
1 tablespoon coconut flour
1 tablespoon cilantro, chopped

Directions:
In a bowl, add crab meat, mustard, mayonnaise, coconut flour, egg, cilantro, salt, and pepper; mix to combine. Make patties out of the mixture. Melt coconut oil in a skillet over medium heat. Add crab patties and cook for 2-3 minutes per side. Remove to kitchen paper. Serve.

Nutrition:
calories 316 | fat 24.3g | protein 15.2g | carbs 1.8g | net carb: 1.5g | fiber 0.3g

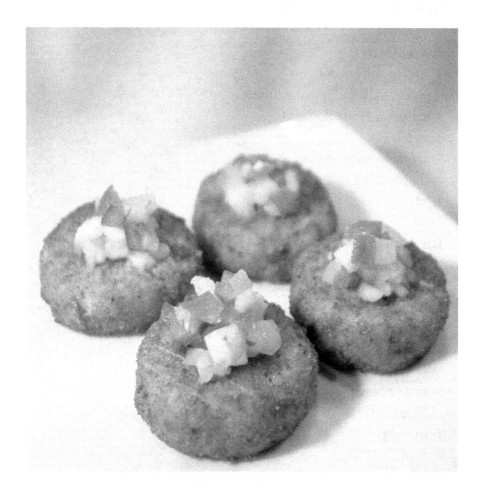

Salads

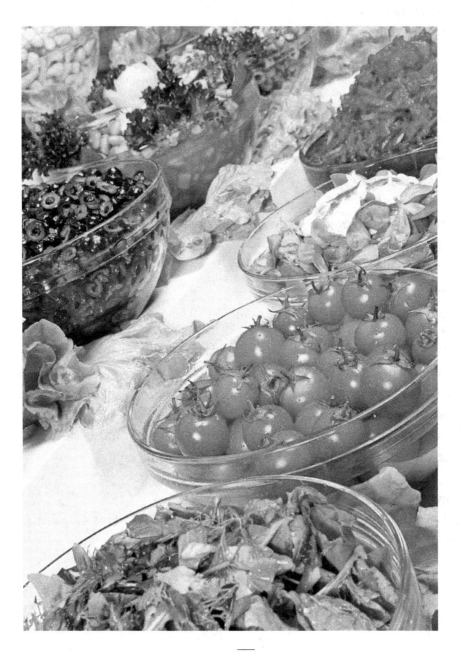

Spicy Leek and Green Cabbage Salad

Preparation time: 15 minutes
Cooking time: 40 minutes
Servings: 4

Ingredients:
3 tablespoons extra-virgin olive oil
1 medium-sized leek, chopped
½ pound (227 g) green cabbage, shredded
½ teaspoon caraway seeds
Sea salt, to taste
4-5 black peppercorns 1 garlic clove, minced
1 teaspoon yellow mustard
1 tablespoon balsamic vinegar
½ teaspoon Sriracha sauce

Directions:
Drizzle 2 tablespoons of the olive oil over the leek and cabbage;
sprinkle with caraway seeds, salt, black peppercorns.
Roast in the preheated oven at 420ºF (216ºC) for 37 to 40 minutes.
Place the roasted mixture in a salad bowl.
Toss with the remaining tablespoon of olive oil garlic, mustard,
vinegar, and Sriracha sauce. Serve immediately and enjoy!

Nutrition:
calories 116 | fat 10.1g | protein 1.0g | carbs 6.5g | net carbs 4.7g |
fiber 1.8g

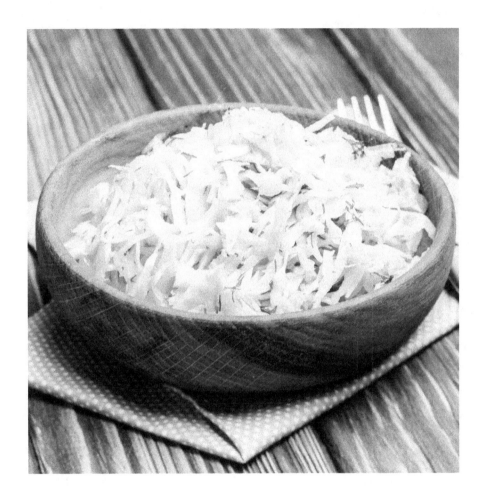

Marinated Pork and Veg Salad

Preparation time: 15 minutes
Cooking time: 15 minutes
Servings: 6

Ingredients:
¼ cup rice vinegar
¼ cup rice wine
¼ cup coconut aminos
1 tablespoon brown mustard
jalapeño pepper, chopped
garlic cloves, pressed
2 tablespoons olive oil
2 pounds (907 g) pork rib chops
Flaky sea salt and ground black pepper, to taste
½ teaspoon celery seeds
6 cups lettuce, torn into small pieces
1 bell pepper, deseeded and sliced
1 cucumber, sliced
1 tomato, sliced
4 scallions, chopped
½ lemon, juiced
½ cup sour cream, for garnish

Directions:

Place the vinegar, wine, coconut aminos, mustard, jalapeño pepper, garlic, and pork in a ceramic dish. Cover and let it marinate for 2 hours in your refrigerator. Heat the olive oil in an oven-safe pan over a medium-high flame. Discard the marinade and cook the pork rib chops for 3 to 5 minutes. Flip them over using a pair of tongs. Cook an additional 4 minutes or until a good crust is formed. Sprinkle with salt, black pepper, and celery seeds. Then, bake the pork rib chops in the preheated oven for 10 minutes until an instantread thermometer reads 145°F (63°C). Shred the pork rib chops and reserve. Add the lettuce, bell pepper, cucumber, tomato, and scallions to a salad bowl. Top with the shredded pork, drizzle lemon juice over everything and garnish with sour cream. Enjoy!

Nutrition:

calories 297 | fat 14.1g | protein 35.2g | carbs 6.0g | net carb: 4.5g | fiber 1.5g

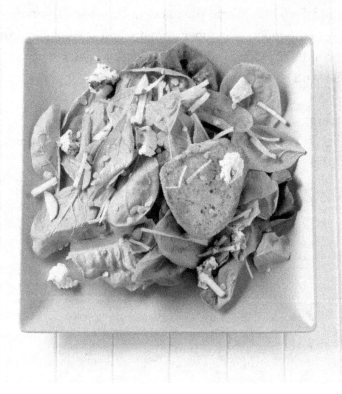

Roasted Asparagus and Cherry Tomato Salad

Preparation time: 15 minutes
Cooking time: 20 minutes
Servings: 3

Ingredients:
1 pound (454 g) asparagus, trimmed
¼ teaspoon ground black pepper
Flaky salt, to season
3 tablespoons sesame seeds
1 tablespoon Dijon mustard
½ lime, freshly squeezed
3 tablespoons extra-virgin olive oil
2 garlic cloves, minced
1 tablespoon fresh tarragon, snipped
1 cup cherry tomatoes, sliced

Directions:

Start by preheating your oven to 400°F (205°C). Spritz a roasting pan with nonstick cooking spray.

Roast the asparagus for about 13 minutes, turning the spears over once or twice. Sprinkle with salt, pepper, and sesame seeds; roast an additional 3 to 4 minutes.

To make the dressing, whisk the Dijon mustard, lime juice, olive oil, and minced garlic.

Chop the asparagus spears into bite-sized pieces and place them in a nice salad bowl. Add the tarragon and tomatoes to the bowl; gently toss to combine.

Dress your salad and serve at room temperature. Enjoy!

Nutrition:

calories 160 | fat 12.4g | protein 5.7g | carbs 6.2g | net carbs 2.2g | fiber 4.0g

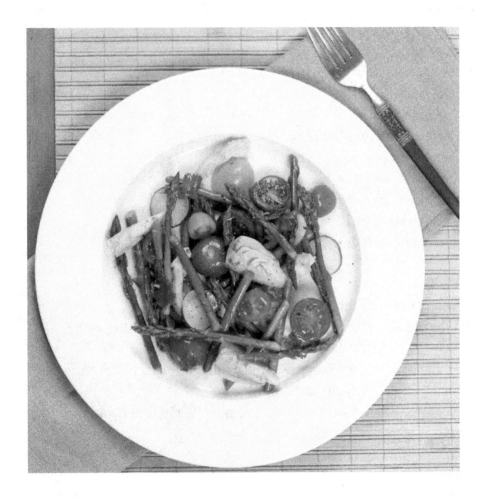

Chicken and Sunflower Seed Salad

Preparation time: 15 minutes
Cooking time: 15 minutes
Servings: 3

Ingredients:
chicken breast, skinless
¼ mayonnaise
¼ cup sour cream
tablespoons Cottage cheese, room temperature
Salt and black pepper, to taste
¼ cup sunflower seeds, hulled and roasted
½ avocado, peeled and cubed
½ teaspoon fresh garlic, minced
2 tablespoons scallions, chopped

Directions:
Bring a pot of well-salted water to a rolling boil.
Add the chicken to the boiling water; now, turn off the heat, cover, and let the chicken stand in the hot water for 15 minutes.
Then, drain the water; chop the chicken into bite-sized pieces. Add the remaining ingredients and mix well.
Place in the refrigerator for at least one hour. Serve well chilled. Enjoy!

Nutrition:
calories 401 | fat 35.2g | protein 16.2g | carbs 5.7g | net carbs 2.9g | fiber 2.8g

Spanish Chicken and Pepper Salad

Preparation time: 10 minutes
Cooking time: 15 minutes
Servings: 6

Ingredients:
1½ pounds (680 g) chicken breasts
½ cup dry white wine
onion, chopped
Spanish peppers, deveined and chopped
Spanish naga chili pepper, chopped
garlic cloves, minced
2 cups arugula
¼ cup mayonnaise
1 tablespoon balsamic vinegar
1 tablespoon stone-ground mustard

Directions:
Sea salt and freshly ground black pepper, to season
Place the chicken breasts in a saucepan. Add the wine to the
saucepan and cover the chicken with water. Bring to a boil over
medium-high heat. Reduce to a simmer and cook partially covered
for 10 to 14 minutes (an instant-read thermometer should register
165°F (74°C)). Transfer the chicken from the poaching liquid to a
cutting board; cut into bite-sized pieces and transfer to a salad bowl.
Add the remaining ingredients to the salad bowl and gently stir to
combine. Serve well chilled.

Nutrition:
calories: 280 | fat: 16.2g | protein: 27.2g | carbs: 4.9g | net carbs: 4.0g
| fiber: 0.9g

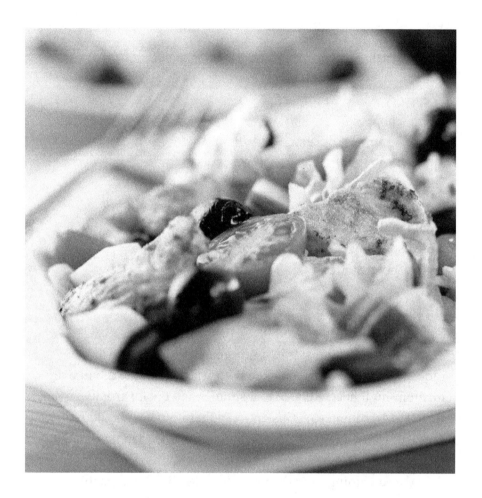

Soups

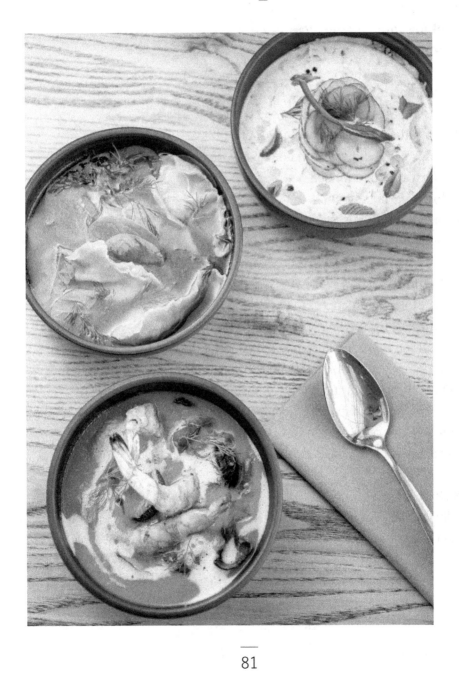

Garlicky Coconut Milk and Tomato Soup

Preparation time: 15 minutes
Cooking time: 30 minutes
Servings: 6

Ingredients:
6 cups vegetable broth
½ cup full-fat unsweetened coconut milk
1½ cups canned diced tomatoes
1 yellow onion, chopped
3 cloves garlic, chopped
1 teaspoon Italian seasoning
1 bay leaf

Directions:
Pinch of salt and pepper, to taste
Fresh basil, for serving
Add all the ingredients minus the coconut milk and fresh basil to a stockpot over medium heat and bring to a boil. Reduce to a simmer and cook for 30 minutes.
Remove the bay leaf, and then use an immersion blender to blend the soup until smooth. Stir in the coconut milk.
Garnish with fresh basil and serve.

Nutrition:
calories 105 | fat 6.9g | protein 6.1g | carbs 5.8g | net carbs 4.8g | fiber 1.0g

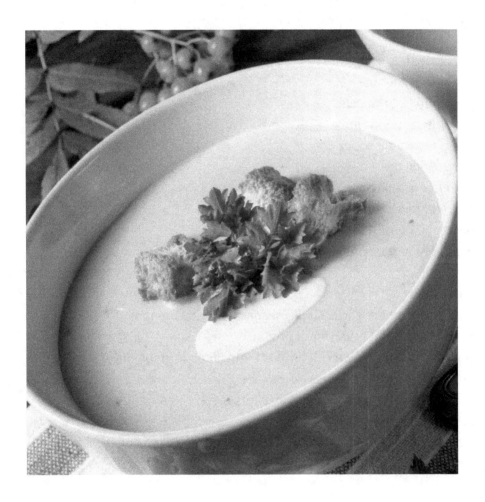

Creamy Mixed Seafood Soup

Preparation Time: 15 minutes
Cooking Time: 15 minutes
Servings: 4

Ingredients:
 tbsp. avocado oil
garlic cloves, minced
3/4 tbsp. almond flour
1 cup vegetable broth
1 tsp. dried dill
1 lb. frozen mixed seafood
Salt and black pepper to taste
tbsp. plain vinegar
cups cooking creamFresh dill leaves to garnish

Directions:
Heat oil sauté the garlic for 30 seconds or until fragrant.
Stir in the almond flour until brown.
Mix in the vegetable broth until smooth and stir in the dill, seafood
mix, salt, and black pepper.
Bring the soup to a boil and then simmer for 3 to 4 minutes or until
the seafood cooks.
Add the vinegar, cooking cream, and stir well. Garnish with dill,
serve.

Nutrition:
Calories 361 | Fat: 12.4g | Fiber: 8.5g | Carbohydrates:3.9 g |
Protein: 11.7g

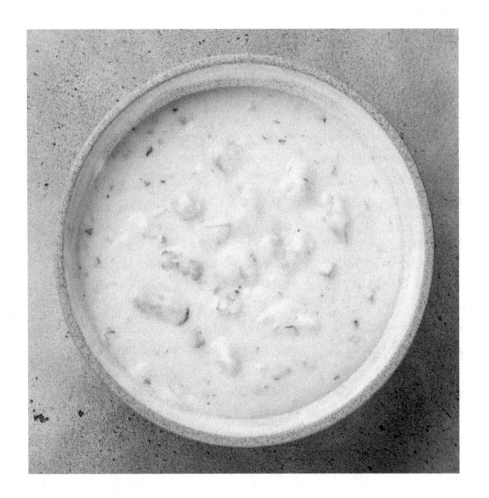

Keto Cabbage Soup

Preparation Time: 10 minutes
Cooking Time: 30 minutes
Servings: 6

Ingredients:
1/4 cup onion, diced
1 clove garlic, minced
1 tsp. cumin
1 head cabbage, chopped
1 1/4 cup canned diced tomatoes
5 oz. canned green chilis
4 cups vegetable stock Salt and pepper to taste

Directions:
Heat a heavy stockpot over medium-high heat. Add the onions and sauté for 5- 7 minutes more. Add the garlic and sauté for one more minute.
Bring this in to a low simmer and cook until the vegetables are tender about 30 minutes. And add water, if necessary, during cooking.
Transfer to serving bowls and serve hot.

Nutrition:
Calories 131 | Fat 4.3g | Fiber 5.9g | Carbohydrates 1.2 g | Protein 5.1g

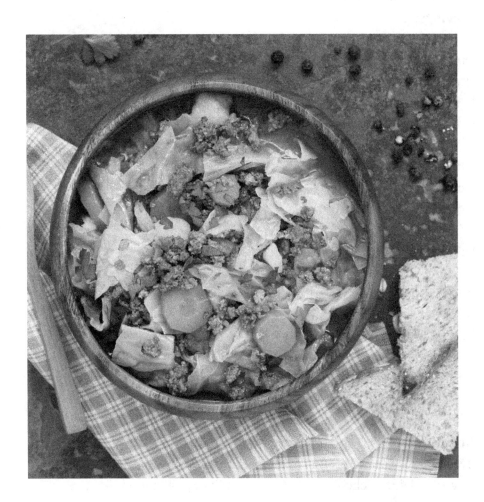

Yogurt Soup

Preparation time: 10 minutes
Cooking time: 5 hours
Servings: 4

Ingredients:
1 cup Greek yogurt
½ teaspoon dried mint
½ teaspoon ground black pepper
1 onion, diced
1 tablespoon coconut oil
3 cups chicken stock
7 oz. chicken fillet, chopped

Directions
Melt the coconut oil in the skillet.
Add onion and roast it until light brown.
After this, transfer the roasted onion in the slow cooker.
Add dried mint, ground black pepper, chicken stock, and chicken fillet.
Add Greek yogurt and carefully mix the soup ingredients.
Close the lid and cook the soup on High for 5 hours.

Nutrition:
180 calories | 20.2g protein | 5.3g carbohydrates | 8.6g fat | 0.7g fiber | 47mg cholesterol | 633mg sodium | 247mg potassium.

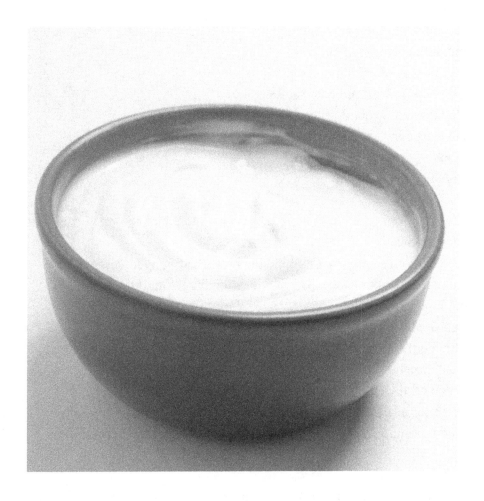

Egg Drop Soup

Preparation Time: 5 minutes
Cooking Time: 10 minutes
Servings: 2

Ingredients:
4 cups chicken broth
teaspoon pink Himalayan sea salt
1/2 teaspoon ground ginger
1/2 teaspoon toasted sesame oil
Pinch of ground white pepper
large eggs
1 scallion

Directions:
In a medium saucepan, combine the broth, salt, ginger, sesame oil, and white pepper. Cook over medium-high heat until the soup is boiling.
In a small bowl, lightly beat the eggs.
Stirring the soup in a circular motion, slowly drizzle the beaten egg into the center of the vortex.
When all the egg is mixed in, stop stirring.
Cook for an additional 2 minutes, until the egg is cooked through, then pour into 2 bowls, sprinkle with the scallions, and serve.

Nutrition:
Calories 121 | Fat 5.1g | Fiber 2.9g |Carbohydrates 1.2 g |
Protein: 10g

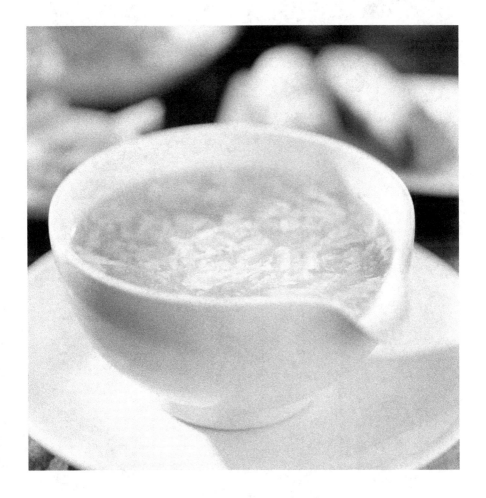

Snacks and Appetizers

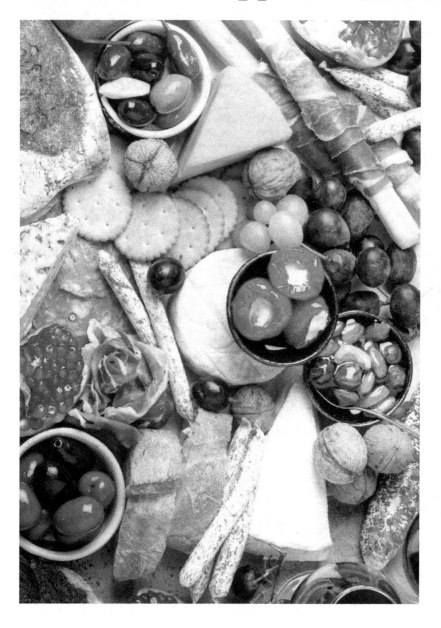

Tex-Mex Queso Dip

Preparation Time: 5 minutes
Cooking Time: 10 minutes
Servings: 6

Ingredients:
1/2 cup of coconut milk
1/2 jalapeño pepper, seeded and diced
teaspoon minced garlic
1/2 teaspoon onion powder
ounces goat cheese
6 ounces sharp Cheddar cheese, shredded
1/4 teaspoon cayenne pepper

Directions:
Preheat a pot then add the coconut milk, jalapeño, garlic, and onion powder.
Simmer then whisk in the goat cheese until smooth.
Add the Cheddar cheese and cayenne and whisk until the dip is thick, 30 seconds to 1 minute.

Nutrition:
Calories 149 | Fat 12.1g |Fiber 3.1g | Carbohydrates 5.1 g | Protein 4.2g

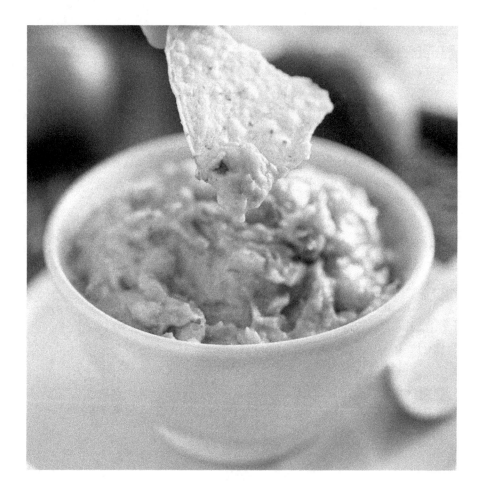

Cheese and Shrimp Stuffed Celery

Preparation time: 10 minutes
Cooking time: 5 minutes
Servings: 6

Ingredients:
5 ounces (142 g) shrimp
10 ounces (283 g) cottage cheese, at room temperature
4 ounces (113 g) Coby cheese, shredded
2 scallions, chopped
1 teaspoon yellow mustard
Sea salt, to taste
½ teaspoon oregano
6 stalks celery, cut into halves

Directions:
Gently pat the shrimp dry with a paper towel.
Cook the shrimp in a lightly greased skillet over medium-high heat for 2 minutes; turn them over and cook for a further 2 minutes.
Chop the shrimp and transfer to a mixing bowl. Add in the cheese, scallions, mustard, and spices. Mix to combine well.
Divide the shrimp mixture between the celery stalks and serve. Bon appétit!

Nutrition:
calories 127 | fat 6.1g | protein 13.4g | carbs 4.2g | net carbs 3.7g | fiber 0.5g

Herbed Cheese Chips

Preparation Time: 15 minutes
Cooking Time: 15 minutes
Servings: 8

Ingredients:
3 tbsp. coconut flour
1/2 C. strong cheddar cheese, grated and divided
1/4 C. Parmesan cheese, grated
2 tbsp. butter, melted
1 organic egg
1 tsp. fresh thyme leaves, minced

Directions:
Preheat the oven to 3500 F. Line a large baking sheet with
parchment paper.
In a bowl, place the coconut flour, 1/4 C. of grated cheddar,
Parmesan, butter, and egg and mix until well combined.
Make eight equal-sized balls from the mixture.
Arrange the balls onto a prepared baking sheet in a single layer about
2-inch apart.
Form into flat discs.
Sprinkle each disc with the remaining cheddar, followed by thyme.
Bake for around 15 minutes.

Nutrition:
Calories 101 | Fat 6.5g | Fiber 1.4g | Carbohydrates 1.2g |
Protein 3.1g

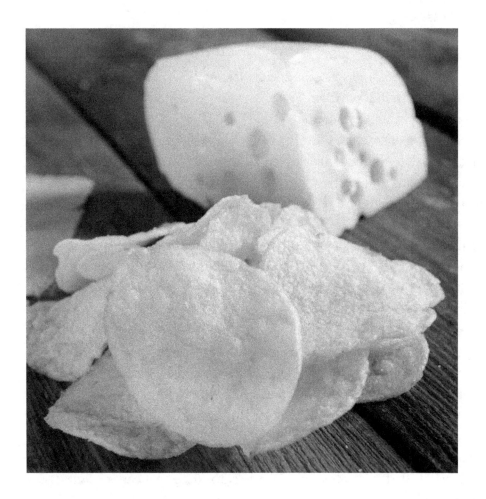

Wrapped Asparagus with Prosciutto

Preparation time: 15 minutes
Cooking time: 20 minutes
Servings: 6

Ingredients:

1½ pounds (680 g) asparagus spears, trimmed
1 teaspoon shallot powder
½ teaspoon granulated garlic
½ teaspoon paprika
Kosher salt and ground black pepper, to taste
1 tablespoon sesame oil
10 slices prosciutto

Directions:

Toss the asparagus spears with the shallot powder, garlic, paprika, salt, and black pepper. Drizzle sesame oil all over the asparagus spears.

Working one at a time, wrap a prosciutto slice on each asparagus spear; try to cover the entire length of the asparagus spear.

Place the wrapped asparagus spears on a parchment-lined roasting pan. Bake in the preheated oven at 390°F (199°C) for about 18 minutes or until thoroughly cooked. Bon appétit!

Nutrition:

calories 120 | fat 6.5g | protein 10.1g | carbs 6.2g | net carbs 3.2g | fiber 3.0g

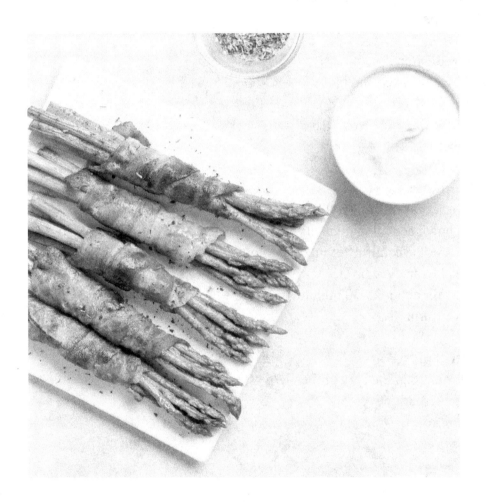

Cauliflower Poppers

Preparation Time: 20 minutes
Cooking Time: 30 minutes
Servings: 4

Ingredients:
4 C. cauliflower florets
2 tsp. olive oil
1/4 tsp. chili powder
Pepper and salt

Directions:
Preheat the oven to 4500 F. Grease a roasting pan.
In a bowl, add all ingredients and toss to coat well.
Transfer the cauliflower mixture into a prepared roasting pan and
spread in an even layer.
Roast for about 25-30 minutes.
Serve warm.

Nutrition:
Calories 102 | Fat 8.5g | Fiber 4.7g | Carbohydrates 2.1 g |
Protein: 4.2g

Chicken and Spinach Meatballs

Preparation time: 15 minutes
Cooking time: 25 minutes
Servings: 10

Ingredients:
1½ pounds (680 g) ground chicken
8 ounces (227 g) Parmigiano-Reggiano cheese, grated
1 teaspoon garlic, minced
1 tablespoon Italian seasoning mix 1 egg, whisked
8 ounces (227 g) spinach, chopped
½ teaspoon mustard seeds
Sea salt and ground black pepper, to taste
½ teaspoon paprika

Directions:
Mix the ingredients until everything is well incorporated.
Now, shape the meat mixture into 20 meatballs. Transfer your meatballs to a baking sheet and brush them with a nonstick cooking oil.
Bake in the preheated oven at 390°F (199°C) for about 25 minutes or until golden brown. Serve with cocktail sticks and enjoy!

Nutrition:
calories 210 | fat 12.4g | protein 19.4g | carbs 4.5g | net carbs 4.0g | fiber 0.5g

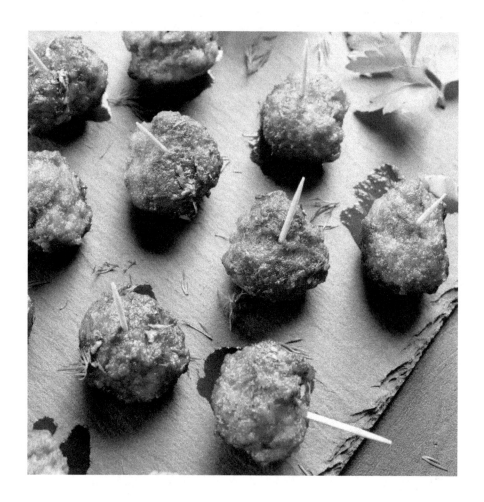

Dessert

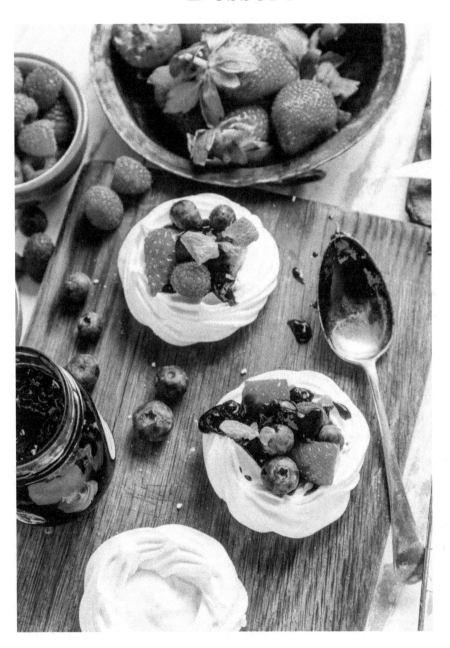

Pecan Pralines

Preparation time: 5 minutes
Cooking time: 15 minutes
Makes: 18 clusters

Ingredients:
4 tablespoons (½ stick) unsalted butter, at room temperature
¼ cup granulated erythritol–monk fruit blend
1½ cups pecan halves
½ teaspoon salt
2 tablespoons heavy whipping cream

Directions:
Line the baking sheet with parchment paper and set aside.
In the skillet, melt the butter over medium-high heat. Using the
silicone spatula, stir in the erythritol–monk fruit blend and combine
well, making sure to dissolve the sugar in the butter. Stir in the pecan
halves and salt.
Once the pecans are completely covered in the glaze, add the heavy
cream and quickly stir. When the heavy cream bubbles and
evaporates, remove from the heat immediately. Quickly spoon the
clusters of 4 to 5 pecan halves each onto the prepared baking sheet
and allow to fully cool and set, 15 to 20 minutes, before enjoying.
Store leftovers in an airtight container on the counter or in the
refrigerator for up 5 days.
Nutrition:
 (1 Cluster) calories:86 | fat 9.0g | protein 1.0g | carbs 1.0g |
net carbs 0g | fiber 1.0g

Coconut Cheesecake

Preparation Time: 15 minutes
Cooking Time: 25 minutes
Servings: 12

Ingredients:
Crust:
 egg whites
1/4 cup erythritol
cups desiccated coconut
1 tsp. coconut oil 1/4 cup melted butter

Filling:
 3 tbsp. lemon juice
6 ounces raspberries
2 cups erythritol
1 cup whipped cream
Zest of 1 lemon 24 ounces cream cheese

Directions:
Line the pan with parchment paper. Preheat oven to 350°F and mix all crust ingredients. Pour the crust into the pan. Bake for about 25 minutes; let cool.
Whisk the cream cheese in a container. Add the lemon juice, zest, and erythritol. Fold in whipped cream mixture. Fold in the raspberries gently. Spoon the filling into the crust. Place in the fridge for 4 hours.

Nutrition:
Calories 214 | Fat 11.4g | Fiber 8.4g | Carbohydrates 5.4g |
Protein: 9.1g

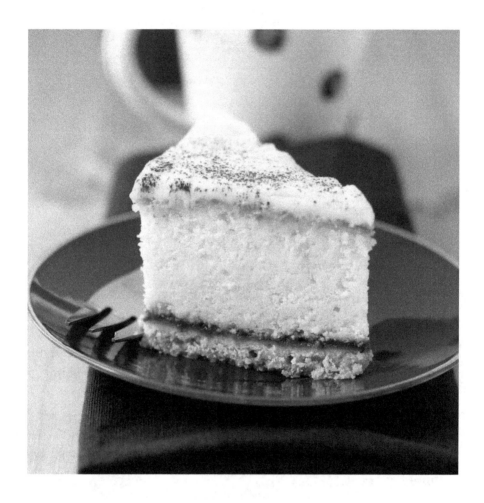

Chocolate Almond Bark

Preparation time: 10 minutes
Cooking time: 0 minutes
Makes: 15 pieces

Ingredients:
¾ cup coconut oil
¼ cup confectioners' erythritol–monk fruit blend; less sweet: 3 tablespoons
3 tablespoons dark cocoa powder
½ cup slivered almonds
¾ teaspoon almond extract

Directions:
Line the baking pan with parchment paper and set aside.
In the microwave-safe bowl, melt the coconut oil in the microwave in 10-second intervals.
In the medium bowl, whisk together the melted coconut oil, confectioners' erythritol–monk fruit blend, and cocoa powder until fully combined. Stir in the slivered almonds and almond extract.
Pour the mixture into the prepared baking pan and spread evenly. Put the pan in the freezer for about 20 minutes, or until the chocolate bark is solid.
Once the chocolate bark is solid, break apart into 15 roughly even pieces to serve.
Store the chocolate bark in an airtight container in the freezer. Allow to slightly thaw about 5 minutes before eating. Thaw only what you will be eating.

Nutrition: (1 Pieces) calories 118 | fat 13.0g | protein 1.0g | carb: 1.0g | net carbs 0g | fiber

Raspberry Tart

Preparating time: 20 minutes
Cooking tima: 4 hours
Servings: 6

Ingredients:
1 cup raspberries
4 tablespoons coconut flour
4 tablespoons butter
3 tablespoons Erythritol
1 teaspoon vanilla extract 1 teaspoon ground ginger

Directions:
Combine butter, coconut flour, ground ginger, and vanilla extract.
Knead the dough.
Cover the bottom of the slow cooker with parchment.
Place the dough in the slow cooker and flatten it to the shape of a pie crust.
Place the raspberries over the piecrust and sprinkle with Erythritol.
Cook the tart for 4 hours on High.
Serve the cooked tart chilled.

Nutrition:
calories 101 | fat 7.9 | fiber 1.5 | carbs 14.2 | protein 0.9

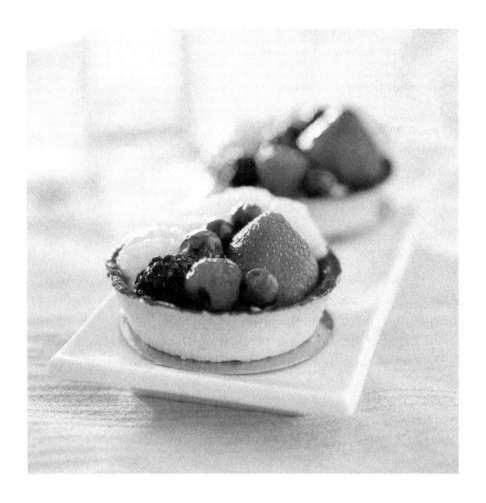

Kombucha Cake

Preparation time: 25 minutes
Cooking time: 3 hours
Servings: 8

Ingredients:
cup almond flour
¼ cup coconut flour
tablespoons Erythritol
¼ teaspoon baking powder
eggs, beaten
2 tablespoons kombucha
¾ teaspoon salt

Directions:
Mix the almond flour and coconut flour.
Add the Erythritol and baking powder.
Add the kombucha and salt and stir the mixture.
Add the beaten eggs and stir the batter until smooth.
Place the batter in the slow cooker and cook for 3 hours on High.
Chill the cooked cake slightly.
Enjoy!

Nutrition:
calories 59 | fat 3.8 | fiber 1.9 | carbs 7.2 | protein 3

Drinks

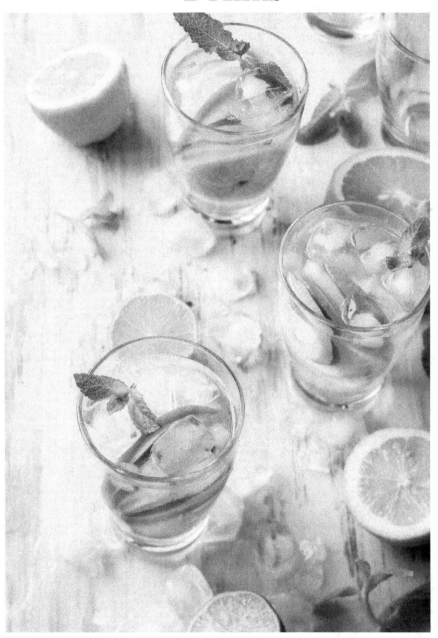

Bulletproof Coffee

Preparation Time: 5 minutes
Cooking Time: 0 minutes
Servings: 1

Ingredients:
11/2 cups hot coffee
2 tablespoons MCT oil powder or Bulletproof Brain Octane Oil
2 tablespoons butter or ghee

Directions:
Pour the hot coffee into the blender.
Add the oil powder and butter, and blend until thoroughly mixed and frothy.
Pour into a large mug and enjoy.

Nutrition:
Calories 245 | Fat 9.4g | Fiber 4.2 g | Carbohydrates:1.2 g | Protein 2.3g

Raita

Preparation time: 8 minutes
Cooking time: 0 minutes
Makes: 1 cup

Ingredients:
⅓ cup full-fat Greek yogurt
⅓ cup full-fat sour cream
¼ cup finely chopped cucumbers
1 tablespoon chopped fresh cilantro
1 tablespoon chopped fresh mint
1 teaspoon granulated erythritol
1 teaspoon minced red onions
¼ teaspoon ground cumin

Direction:
Place all of the ingredients in a small bowl and mix well. Serve immediately or store in an airtight container in the refrigerator for up to 3 days.

Nutrition:
calories 30 | fat 2.1g | protein 0.9g | carbs 1.0g | net carbs 1.0g | fiber 0g

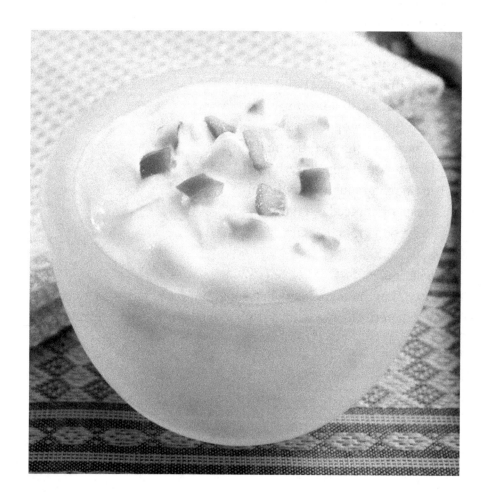

Raspberry Coulis

Preparation time: 3 minutes
Cooking time: 5 minutes
Makes: 1½ cups

Ingredients:
2 cups fresh or frozen red raspberries
2 tablespoons granulated erythritol

Direction:
Combine the raspberries and sweetener in a small saucepan and cook over medium heat for 5 minutes, or until bubbling.
Blend with an immersion blender for 30 seconds or until liquefied, then pour the sauce through a fine-mesh strainer to remove any seed fragments. Let cool before using.
Store in an airtight container in the refrigerator for up to 1 week or in the freezer for up to 3 months.

Nutrition:
calories 13 | fat 0g | protein 0g | carbs 2.6g | net carbs 1.0g | fiber 1.6g

BBQ Sauce

Preparation time: 8 minutes
Cooking time: 0 minutes
Makes: ¾ cup

Ingredients:
½ cup reduced-sugar ketchup, store-bought or homemade
2 tablespoons apple cider vinegar
2 tablespoons granulated erythritol
1 tablespoon filtered water
1½ teaspoons ground allspice
1½ teaspoons ground mustard powder
1 teaspoon blackstrap molasses (optional; see note)
½ teaspoon liquid smoke
½ teaspoon onion powder
½ teaspoon Worcestershire sauce
¼ teaspoon ground cloves
¼ teaspoon xanthan gum (optional, to thicken)

Directions:
Place all of the ingredients in a medium-sized bowl and whisk together. Store in an airtight container in the refrigerator for up to 2 weeks.

Nutrition:
calories 15 | fat 0g | protein 0g | carbs 2.8g | net carbs 2.8g | fiber 0g

Tomato and Bacon Dressing

Preparation time: 8 minutes
Cooking time: 0 minutes
Makes: ¾ cup

Ingredients:
¼ cup sugar-free mayonnaise
5 cherry tomatoes
3 slices bacon, cooked and chopped
clove garlic, peeled
tablespoons chopped fresh parsley
½ teaspoon granulated erythritol
¼ teaspoon kosher salt
⅛ teaspoon ground black pepper

Directions:
Place all of the ingredients in a small blender and blend until mostly smooth. Store in an airtight container in the refrigerator for up to 1 week.

Nutrition:
calories 95 | fat 10.0g | protein 2.0g | carbs 1.0g | net carbs 1.0g | fiber 0

Other keto Diet

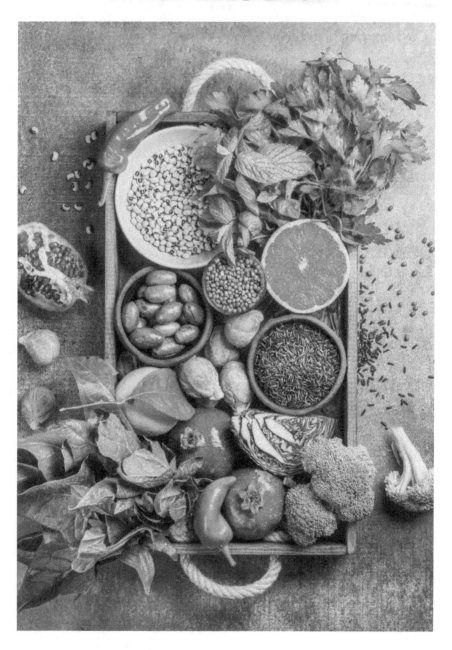

Rosemary Turkey Sausage Egg Muffins

Preparation time: 5 minutes
Cooking time: 15 minutes
Servings: 3

Ingredients:
1 teaspoon butter
6 eggs
Salt and black pepper, to taste
½ teaspoon dried rosemary
1 cup pecorino romano cheese, grated
3 turkey sausages, chopped

Directions:
Preheat oven to 400°F (205°C) and grease muffin cups with cooking spray.
In a skillet over medium heat add the butter and cook the turkey sausages for
4-5 minutes.
Beat 3 eggs with a fork. Add in sausages, cheese, and seasonings. Divide
between the muffin cups and bake for 4 minutes. Crack in an egg to each of
the cups. Bake for an additional 4 minutes. Allow cooling before serving.

Nutrition:
calories: 422 | fat: 34.2g | protein: 26.4g | carbs: 2.1g | net carbs: 2.1g |
fiber: 0g

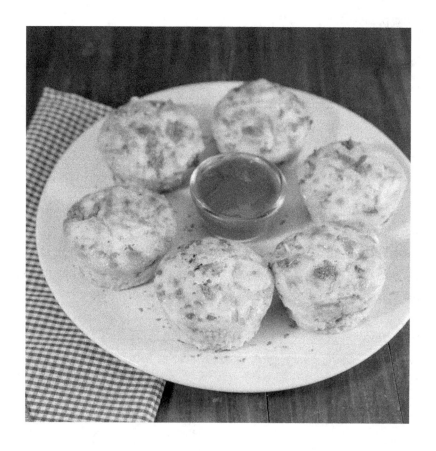

Queso Fresco Avocado Salsa

Preparation time: 5 minutes
Cooking time: 0 minutes
Servings: 4

Ingredients:
2 tomatoes, diced
3scallions, chopped
1 poblano pepper, chopped
garlic clove, minced
ripe avocados, peeled, pitted and diced
tablespoon extra-virgin olive oil
tablespoons fresh lime juice
Sea salt and ground black pepper, to season
¼ cup queso fresco, crumbled

Directions:
Place the tomatoes, scallions, poblano pepper, garlic and avocado in a serving bowl. Drizzle olive oil and lime juice over everything.
Season with salt and black pepper.
To serve, top with crumbled queso fresco and enjoy!

Nutrition:
calories: 189 | fat: 16.0g | protein: 3.6g | carbs: 6.9g | net carbs: 2.7g | fiber: 4.2g

Curried Shrimp and Cabbage

Preparation time: 10 minutes
Cooking time: 6 hours
Servings: 4

Ingredients:
4 cups cabbage, shredded
cup onion, sliced thin
cloves garlic, crushed and minced
1 tablespoon curry powder
1 teaspoon salt
1 teaspoon black pepper
1 cup chicken or fish stock
1 cup coconut milk
1 pound shrimp, cleaned and deveined
¼ cup butter, melted ¼ cup full fat yogurt
¼ cup fresh cilantro, chopped

Directions:
Place the cabbage, onion, garlic, curry powder, salt, and black
pepper in a slow cooker and toss to mix. Next, add the chicken or
fish stock and coconut milk. Cover and cook on high for 4 hours.
Remove the lid from the slow cooker and add the shrimp, melted
butter, and yogurt. Cover and cook an additional 10-15 minutes, or
until the shrimp is cooked through. Garnish with fresh cilantro
before serving.

Nutrition:
Calories 274.7 | Fat 14.8 g | Carbs 9.7 g | Protein 26.3 g |
Dietary Fiber 3.3 g | Sugars 1 g

Hazelnut Haddock Bake

Preparation time: 15 minutes
Cooking time: 25 minutes
Servings: 4

Ingredients:
1 tablespoon butter
1 shallot, sliced
pound (454 g) haddock fillet
eggs, hard-boiled, chopped
½ cup water
tablespoons hazelnut flour
2 cups sour cream
1 tablespoon parsley, chopped
½ cup pork rinds, crushed
1 cup Mozzarella cheese, grated
Salt and black pepper to taste

Directions:
Melt butter in a saucepan over medium heat and sauté the shallots for about 3 minutes. Reduce the heat to low and stir the hazelnut flour into it to form a roux. Cook the roux to be golden brown and stir in the sour cream until the mixture is smooth. Season with salt and pepper, and stir in the parsley. Spread the haddock fillet in a greased baking dish, sprinkle the eggs on top, and spoon the sauce over. In a bowl, mix the pork rinds with the Mozzarella cheese, and sprinkle it over the sauce. Bake in the oven for 20 minutes at 370°F (188°C) until the top is golden and the sauce and cheese are bubbly.
Nutrition:
calories: 786 | fat: 56.9g | protein: 64.9g | carbs: 9.5g | net carbs: 8.4g | fiber: 1.1g

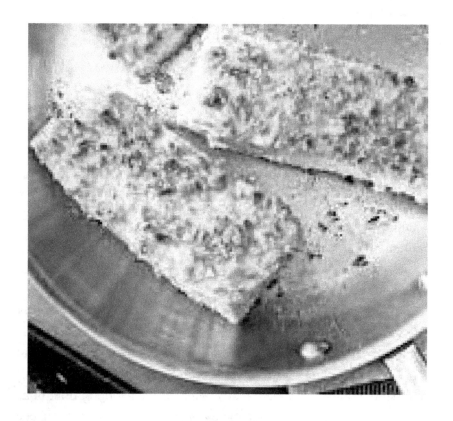

White Tuna Patties

Preparation time: 5 minutes
Cooking time: 20 minutes
Servings: 3

Ingredients:
2 large eggs
tablespoon fresh lemon juice¼ cup grated Parmesan cheese
¼ cup golden flaxseed meal
tablespoons chopped fresh parsley
2 teaspoons Old Bay seasoning
1 (12-ounce / 340-g) can white tuna, in water
¼ cup finely chopped onions
¼ teaspoon salt
¼ cup avocado oil, for frying
Lemon wedges, for serving (optional)

Directions:
In a bowl, beat the eggs with the lemon juice.
Stir in the Parmesan cheese, flaxseed meal, parsley, and Old Bay
seasoning. Drain the tuna well, removing as much of the water as
possible. Add the drained tuna and onions to the Parmesan mixture
and mix well. Season with salt and pepper to taste. Shape the tuna
mixture into 6 patties. Heat the oil in a large skillet over medium
heat. When hot, add half of the patties and fry until golden brown, 3
to 5 minutes per side, then set on a paper towel–lined dish to soak up
any excess oil. Repeat with the remaining patties.
Serve with lemon wedges, if desired.
Nutrition:
calories: 306 | fat: 18.1g | protein: 30.9g | carbs: 5.0g | net carbs: 2.0g
| fiber: 3.0g

Fried Shrimp Tails

Preparation Time: 10 minutes
Cooking Time: 15 minutes
Servings: 4

Ingredients:
1-pound shrimp tails
1 tablespoon olive oil
teaspoon dried dill
1/2 teaspoon dried parsley
tablespoon coconut flour
1/2 cup heavy cream 1 teaspoon chili flakes

Directions:
Peel the shrimp tails and sprinkle them with the dried dill and dried parsley. Mix the shrimp tails carefully in the mixing bowl. After this, combine the coconut flour, heavy cream, and chili flakes in the separate bowl and whisk it until you get the smooth batter. Then preheat the air fryer to 330 F. Transfer the shrimp tails in the heavy crema batter and stir the seafood carefully. Then spray the air fryer rack and put the shrimp tails there. Cook the shrimp tails for 7 minutes. After this, turn the shrimp tails into another side. Cook the shrimp tails for 7 minutes more. When the seafood is cooked – chill it well. Enjoy!

Nutrition:
Calories: 212 | Fat: 10.1g | Fiber: 8.5g | Carbohydrates:2.6 g | Protein: 5.1g

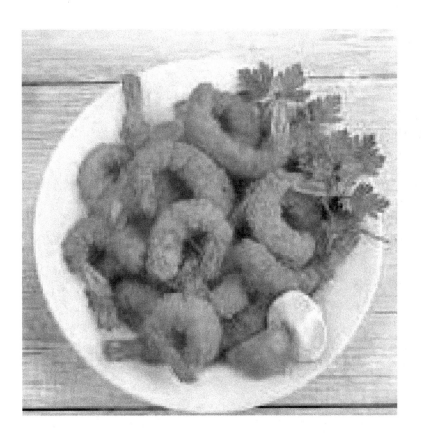

Candied Pecans

Preparation time: 10 minutes
Cooking time: 3 hours
Servings: 4

Ingredients:
1 cup white sugar
1 and ½ tablespoons cinnamon powder
½ cup brown sugar
1 egg white, whisked
4 cups pecans
teaspoons vanilla extract ¼ cup water

Directions:
In a bowl, mix white sugar with cinnamon, brown sugar and vanilla and stir.
Dip pecans in egg white, then in sugar mix and put them in your slow
cooker, also add the water, cover and cook on Low for 3 hours.
Divide into bowls and serve as a snack.

Nutrition
Calories 152 | Fat 4 | Fiber 7 | Carbs 16 | Protein 6

Grilled Mediterranean Veggies

Preparation Time: 10 minutes
Cooking Time: 15 minutes
Servings: 4

Ingredients:
1/4 cup (56 g/2 oz) ghee or butter
small (200 g/7.1 oz) red, orange, or yellow peppers
medium (600 g/21.2 oz) zucchini
1 medium (500 g/17.6 oz) eggplant
1 medium (100 g/3.5 oz) red onion

Directions:
Set the oven to broil to the highest setting. In a small bowl, mix the melted ghee and crushed garlic. Wash all the vegetables. Halve, deseed, and slice the bell peppers into strips. Slice the zucchini widthwise into 1/4-inch (about 1/2 cm) pieces. Wash the eggplant and slice. Quarter each slice into 1/4-inch (about 1/2 cm) pieces. Peel and slice the onion into medium wedges and separate the sections using your hands.
Place the vegetables in a bowl and add the chopped herbs, ghee with garlic, salt, and black pepper. The vegetables must be spread on a baking sheet, ideally on a roasting rack or net, so that the vegetables don't become soggy from the juices.
Put it in the oven and let it cook for about 15 minutes. Be careful not to burn them. When done, the vegetables should be slightly tender but still crisp. Serve with meat dishes or bake with cheese such as feta, mozzarella, or Halloumi.

Nutrition: Calories: 176 | Fat: 4.5g | Fiber: 9.3g |
Carbohydrates: 3.1g | Protein: 5.2 g

Gazpacho Soup

Preparation Time: 25 minutes
Cooking Time: 0 minutes
Servings: 3

Ingredients:
1 large cucumber (to be sliced into chunks)
4 big ripe tomatoes (coarsely chopped)
1/2 bell pepper (any color)
2 cloves of garlic (minced)
1 celery rib (chopped)
1 tablespoon of lemon juice
1/4 tablespoon of celery pepper
1 tablespoon of fresh basil (chopped)
1 tablespoon of fresh parsley (chopped)
Dash black pepper
1/2 tablespoon salt
3 tablespoons of red wine (vinegar/balsamic vinegar)
1/2 sweet onions (quartered)

Directions:

To make the gazpacho, place the cucumber chunks, chopped tomatoes, bell pepper, garlic, celery, lemon juice, and onion in the food processor or blender. You may choose to blend or process in batches if needed. Add the vinegar (red/balsamic), salt, pepper to the blender or food processor and blend or process together until it is smooth or nearly smooth (the texture depends on you)The next step is to pour soup into a serving bowl and stir in the fresh chopped parsley and basil. Cover the serving bowl with plastic wrap or foil or cover it with a plastic wrap and put the bowl inside the refrigerator for about 30 minutes or until when you are set to serve the gazpacho soup. You can decide to add some extra fresh herbs to the soup for presentation as well as some avocado slices or crusty croutons. Serve gazpacho soup with a green salad, some artisanal or homemade bread as a substitute, balsamic vinegar, and olive oil for dipping for a light but a complete meal. Serve and enjoy!

Nutrition:

Calories: 131 | Fat: 9.4g | Fiber: 16.8g | Carbohydrates:2.4 g | Protein: 4.1g

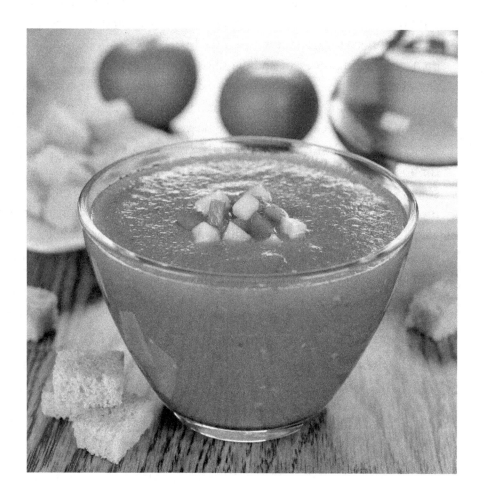

Guacamole and Tomato Soup

Preparation time: 10 minutes
Cooking time: 0 minutes
Servings: 4

Ingredients:
3 cups chicken broth
½ cup heavy cream
2 ripe avocados pitted
½ cup freshly chopped cilantro
1 tomato, chopped
Salt and black pepper, to taste

Directions:
Add all the ingredients to a high-speed blender and blend until creamy.
Chill in the refrigerator for 1 hour before serving.

Nutrition:
calories: 290 | fat: 25.9g | protein: 6.1g | carbs: 10.1g | net carbs: 3.0g | fiber: 7.1g

CPSIA information can be obtained
at www.ICGtesting.com
Printed in the USA
BVHW040611120521
607043BV00002B/694

9 781802 750577